By His Side

By His Side

Life and Love After Stroke

Eileen Steets Quann

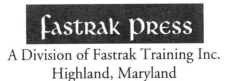

A Division of Fastrak Training Inc.
Highland, Maryland

Published by Fastrak Press, a Division of Fastrak Training Inc.
6595 Castlebay Court, Highland, Maryland 20777-9789
web site http://www.fastrak.com
email fastrakpress@fastrak.com.
First edition

Printed and bound in the United States of America by Signature Book Printing Inc.
www.sbpbooks.com

ISBN 0-9716864-0-8

Library of Congress Control Number: 2002100606

Dedicated to my parents
who taught their children
that they could achieve
whatever they really wanted

To stroke survivors and their families
who work every day toward recovery

and

To my beloved husband John.

Preface

When my husband John had a stroke in 1997, I was incredibly ignorant of the medical issues and terrified of how it would affect our lives. Learning about the technical aspects of his brain injury, though painful to read, meant hours of searching the library, bookstores and the internet. Even as I struggled through the medical information, I longed to read personal stories by survivors and spouses, stories of how they coped and recovered, stories that would offer hope. Today medical information is even more abundant, with dozens of excellent web sites available to help one sift through the technical information, but few memoirs have been published and none–to my knowledge–describe the experience from the perspective of the spouse. I understand now that personal accounts of aphasia are difficult to capture. The stroke survivor is often left without the ability to read, write, speak or understand and the spouse may be as overwhelmed with day to day survival as I was. But in the years following John's stroke, as we dealt head-on with many challenges, I decided to capture our experience. Every stroke is different, every person different, every set of circumstances different. I don't presume that what worked for us would work for others, but I offer this story to readers as a view of stroke and survival from my perspective, as the spouse of a stroke survivor.

The story didn't unfold the way I thought it would when I began. I had intended to write about our experience surviving and recovering from John's stroke, to describe John's physical and mental condition as it changed over time, to detail the process we followed as we dealt with his aphasia. Based on our experience, I wanted to offer encouragement, hope and some practical ideas to others dealing with such a life changing event. What evolved was a story that I had not expected. My mother and a friend who read the initial chapters insisted it was a love story though I fought the idea. As I began to see it through their eyes, I realized that they were right, then debated whether I was willing to share that much of our private life with strangers. Based on the reactions of those who read the manuscript, I now believe that our emotional reaction to John's stroke is as critical to this book as the mental and physical challenges we faced. I have chosen to share this part of my life with others because I have learned that who we have become is far more important than what happened to us.

There are many characters in this book, most of them family members. To reduce the likelihood of confusion for readers, a list of characters appears at the end of the book. Only those who appear on multiple pages throughout the book are listed. I beg your indulgence.

I have much to be thankful for and many who deserve acknowledgment for their role in producing this story. First and foremost, I thank the doctors, nurses and therapists who saved John's life and worked with enthusiasm, kindness and generosity to help him recover. Without them, there would have been no story to tell. If it hadn't been for my sister Andrea Ingram's encouragement to begin this book, this story might still exist only in my mind. It was Nancy Philippi who made me realize that this was a love story, not a story about recovering from a stroke. She generously gave of her time to review chapters, offering valuable criticism and positive feedback, a challenging combination. Roger Jenkin reviewed the manuscript at several stages of its development and suggested critical improvements throughout. Charlotte Mitchum read the manuscript and thought it worthwhile enough to solicit reviews from other prominent people in the field. Without her friendship, encouragement and network of friends, this book might not be in print. My thanks go to the reviewers who took time out of their busy schedule to read a manuscript from an unknown author and write the kind comments that appear on the cover of this book. I am forever grateful to John's and my family who supported us as we survived the initial days and weeks following John's stroke, who read and reread chapters as they were produced, and who encouraged this venture from the start.

Above all, I thank my beloved husband John, who listened with interest each time I read and reread chapters to him, who shared ideas, discussed and suggested improvements, encouraged me throughout this venture, who laughed and cried as he relived the experience, who patiently left me alone to write.

Table of Contents

The Stroke

Saturday, April 12,1997

"We should know in the next 48 hours whether he'll live."
The neurosurgeon had come directly from the operating room to report the outcome of the emergency craniotomy he had just performed on my husband John. I felt both relieved and sickened, so suddenly catapulted into a world beyond my imagination—a world in which I was ignorant of all the rules, certain only that fairness wasn't one of them.

"And then what?" I asked, unable to deal with the possibility that he might die.

"The hemorrhaging was massive. Surgery relieved some of the pressure on John's brain, but I was unable to find the source of the bleeding. We'll be monitoring him to see if there's any more bleeding."

"And then what?" I asked again.

The doctor took a deep breath and spoke slowly, "Your husband is on oxygen. He might not be able to breathe on his own. Stroke victims often have difficulty swallowing and he might be unable to eat solid food. He could also be partially blind."

He paused, as if there was still more bad news, and then continued, cautiously selecting his words. "The bleeding is on the left side of his brain. The left side of the brain controls the motor skills on the right side of his body. It's likely that he'll be paralyzed on his right side—his arm and his leg. The left side of the brain also controls communication. He might not be able to understand you, to speak, read or write."

"But he'll know us, right?" I asked uncertainly.

He hesitated, then said that it was unclear how his memory would be affected.

Denial is a powerful drug. After everything he had said, I still believed that he was describing how John would be for some short time until he recovered. He was alive. He would recover. In my insulated world, people always recovered after an operation.

"How long will it take before he's well again?" I asked. The doctor looked at me strangely, as though I had not understood anything that he had said. I was so unprepared for this, so ignorant, so unable to comprehend it.

Then his look changed to one of understanding. He must have recognized in my voice the sound of denial that pervaded the voices of other spouses, other family members, other patients before me.

"Let's take it one day at a time," he said gently. "Let's see how he does the next couple of days."

It was Saturday afternoon. John had driven to Brooklyn two days earlier to visit his mother while his sister Kathleen, with whom she lived, had gone to Florida. His mother hadn't been well, so John had offered to stay with her. He planned to return home today.

Friday night I was home alone, fixing dinner when the phone rang at about seven. It was John's niece Jeannie.

"Eileen, I don't want you to worry, but Uncle John is having a problem. I'm at Grandma's house. The paramedics are here," she began.

"What kind of a problem?" I asked.

"He had a headache a couple of hours ago. He's very upset now and he's not making much sense. He's having a problem talking. The paramedic needs to talk to you," she said, handing over the phone.

"Mrs. Quann?"

"Yes?"

"Is your husband on any medication?"

"No."

"Does he have high blood pressure?"

"No."

"Does he have any allergies?"

"Not that I know of."

"Does he have any medical problems that we should know about?"

"No, he's in perfect health," I assured him. "Can I speak to him?"

"He can't come to the phone right now. We're taking him to the hospital."

Jeannie came back. She was going with him in the ambulance. Telling me again not to worry, that he would probably be fine, she promised to call as soon as she knew anything.

At that point there wasn't much I could do but wait for her next phone call. Being an optimist, and knowing John to be in excellent health, I thought he was going to the hospital for observation. My initial thoughts were that I would probably have to drive up to New York the next day to bring him home. Then he'd need to schedule an appointment with a doctor for a checkup and maybe some tests. I remember thinking that men were such babies when it came to having a headache and that it would be a pain in the neck to get his car back home.

I called my sister Annie who lived nearby and told her what had happened. John had complained of a headache, and apparently it must have gotten pretty bad. They were taking him to the hospital as a precaution. I would have to go up in the morning to drive him home. If he still had a headache in the morning, the doctor might not want him driving. It sure screwed up the weekend though and I had no idea how we were going to get his car back home.

I was a year older than Annie. We came from a family of seven very independent children, now fanned out over North America, but Annie and I had weathered many storms together. Our first marriages ended about fifteen years ago, and we were each left alone to raise toddlers. It was in those years that we became close, surviving single parenthood together, sharing baby-sitting chores while our children progressed from preschool to elementary school, laughing and crying over tales of hopeless dates, before we both remarried. Now, we talked a lot on the phone and living only a few miles apart, dropped over when we needed to escape from home. She was the natural person to call.

At about the same time, John's sister Kathleen had called home on her drive back from Florida, spoken with her mother and then called me about seven thirty. Kathleen and her son Thomas were in southern Virginia. We agreed that they would spend the night at our house in Maryland, and the three of us would drive up to New York together Saturday morning. At least that solved the car problem.

At ten Jeannie called from the hospital and said that John was sleeping and that the doctor from the emergency room wanted to talk to me. The doctor said that John had been admitted, had been given medication to sedate him and was sleeping. He was having difficulty completing sentences. A CAT scan revealed a small area of bleeding inside his brain. The bleeding could have been caused by hypertension, a defect in the wall, a clot or a tumor. Usually the bleeding stopped on its own, but if it did not, surgery could correct it. Since it could affect his breathing, he was receiving oxygen. They would monitor him overnight and then do more tests, another CAT scan, MRI and an angiogram. The doctor said more, calling it a stroke, but sounded calm.

I was unfamiliar with most of his terminology. How bad can a stroke be? I'd never seen John with anything worse than a cold. But it was probably not a good idea for John to drive back alone tomorrow. I'd never driven John's car. It was a company car. I hated driving in the city. Knowing he could be awfully stubborn, I hoped he wouldn't insist on driving it himself. If he did, it would be a wasted trip for me.

During the night I reassured myself. John was 59 years old and had never been sick. At 5'11", he weighed 170 pounds, jogged a couple of miles every other day, biked 30-50 miles every weekend. His annual physicals indicated that his cholesterol was fine, his blood pressure low. I thought of him as a fitness freak. His diet could have been a health book model. Breakfast was usually fresh squeezed orange juice, muesli or oatmeal, yogurt, cereal, bananas. He often viewed my offer of an omelet on Sunday mornings as a hostile, even homicidal act—murder by cholesterol. John was the only person I knew who could order a sandwich and not touch the potato chips on the side. He was energetic, positive, highly motivated and definitely healthy. People like John didn't suddenly have strokes. The doctor was probably overreacting, being cautious—nobody wants to be sued for malpractice these days. John would be fine in the morning. I fell asleep.

Kathleen, though arriving very late the night before, woke me at five in the morning anxious to get on the road. She suggested I bring some clothes in case I had to spend the night. Reluctantly I acquiesced, still sleepy and secretly hoping this trip wouldn't spill into Sunday. In retrospect, she was probably appalled by my lack of urgency, but we didn't know each other well enough to share such thoughts. I envisioned my role this weekend as the chauffeur.

Thomas, John's nephew, drove. He was a policeman in New York City. He knew how fast he could go—without pushing it. When we stopped on the New Jersey Turnpike for coffee Kathleen called home and came back with a stricken look on her face. She reported that John had gotten worse during the night. We needed to get there as quickly as possible.

Now I was starting to get scared. John's condition was more serious than I had admitted to myself. We drove straight to the hospital, arriving before ten. Mary, John's youngest sister who lived in Manhattan, met us in the lobby, red-eyed and upset and led us to the intensive care unit. I was surprised to see her.

"How's John?" I asked.

"Not good."

"When did you get here?"

"Early this morning."

How did she already know about John? Why was she here early this morning, I wondered. She looked so upset that I was afraid to ask anything else. As we approached the hospital unit, Mary pointed out the doctor from the ICU. Quickly, I walked up to him.

"I'm John Quann's wife. I've just driven up from Maryland to take him home."

He looked at me as if I were crazy. "I don't think you understand. Your husband can't be moved. Have you seen him?"

"No, we just arrived. Where is he?"

The doctor pointed to his room. I don't like hospitals and this place felt old, dark and dreary. I wanted to get out of there as soon as possible. I knew John would too. I approached the door quickly, thinking of what I would say to him, unprepared for what I saw.

Three men, dressed in white were holding John down, trying to give him medication as he lay unconscious and convulsing. He was connected to tubes and monitors. His arms and legs were shaking, his head was twitching and jerking, his eyes were closed. His unshaven face was gray and bloated, the facial muscles slack. He looked like an old man. Was this my John? How could everything have changed so quickly? Just last night they said he had a small bleed. He was supposed to be under observation. Weren't they supposed to be watching him? How could something like this happen? I couldn't believe it. I was terrified. I was furious. Why didn't I know how bad he was? How could this have happened?

The doctor followed me into the room. Earlier that morning, he had contacted a neurosurgeon who was making his patient rounds. The neurosurgeon had seen John and needed to meet with me immediately.

I was too horrified to speak.

"Where's the neurosurgeon?" Mary asked.

She had already seen this. She knew. She had had more time to adjust to seeing John this way. Now I understood her horror. She took my hand and led me into a room crowded with hospital machinery. Dr. Anant entered, introduced himself and pointed to rolling stools where we could sit while he described John's condition. He said there wasn't time to bring in the neurosurgeon who was on call that morning. John had had a catastrophic stroke. They needed to operate immediately. Mary took notes as he spoke. A second CAT scan showed that the bleeding had continued. He held up his fist to demonstrate the size of the area in John's brain that was filled with blood. He talked about drilling a hole in his skull to relieve the pressure in his brain. He talked about the mid-line being shifted.

I didn't understand, or couldn't comprehend everything he said, but I remember the word catastrophic, and I remember the size of his fist. Without the operation he would die. With it, he had a chance.

"What kind of a chance?" I wanted to know. He wouldn't give me odds, but said that they weren't good and repeated that without the operation, John would die. I needed to sign some papers. Who is this guy, I wondered. Is he any good? What choice did I have? Remembering what John looked like, this didn't seem like the time for second opinions. I signed. He left to prepare for surgery.

The wait began. These were surely the longest minutes and hours of my life.

I needed to connect to someone, to tell them about this awful thing. I wanted someone from my family here. My parents lived in Florida. Pop wasn't well and couldn't travel. Mom wouldn't leave him there alone. Using one of the pay phones lined up along the lobby wall, I called my brother Richard in Toronto. Within seconds, my knees buckled, and I slipped to the floor, back against the wall, shaking knees tucked under my chin, sobbing that John might die. He'd had a stroke. It was massive. He was unconscious and convulsing. They were going to operate to try to save his life. He might die! Saying it seemed to make it more real and more frightening.

Richard responded immediately, "Calm down and listen to me. I'll be on the next flight down. Where are you?"

Trying hard to collect my thoughts, I took a deep breath.

"I'm in a hospital in Brooklyn. It's called Maimonides. John's sister Kathleen drove me here. I don't know where it is."

"Don't worry, I'll find it. Everything will be okay. John's strong. If anyone can survive this, John can. Call back in an hour and Cathy will tell you what flight I'm on. I'll be there as soon as I can. Just hang in there."

"Thank you, Richard." I hung up. There had been no hesitation, no doubts, just absolute unquestioning support. He would be here on the next flight. Thank God.

I looked at my watch. Perhaps ten minutes had passed. What next, I thought. The phone was my lifeline. I needed to tell people. They needed to know what I knew. I wanted to call my parents, but I had to calm down. My father was not well. I *had* to calm down. Mom answered the phone.

"Mom, John had a stroke. I'm in New York. John's going into surgery. They don't know if he's going to live," I blurted out. My voice was shaky, but I wasn't crying. This was as calm as I was going to get.

"Eileen?"

"Yeah, mom, it's me."

I repeated and expanded. Richard was coming. No, there was no reason for anyone else to come until we knew more. Yes, I was okay. Yes, there was something she could do, she could call everyone in the family and tell them. Yes, I'd call when I knew more.

I called Annie and fell apart again. She ran a crisis center. She could handle a crisis. She was calm, her words reassuring. John had been in excellent health. He would come out of this okay. I hung up with the promise to keep her informed.

I tried calling my sons David and Sean away at college. No answer either place. Saturday morning, probably still asleep. This wasn't the kind of message to leave on a tape recorder and they wouldn't be able to call me back.

What about medical insurance? I'd never paid much attention to our policy. Neither of us had ever been sick. John was a vice-president at a small engineering services company. His best friend Art, an owner, would help. Art needed to know. The people who worked with John needed to know. Within minutes, there I was again, clutching the pay phone in the lobby, sprawled on the floor, sobbing, choking out the words to tell Art what had happened.

Art was devastated. He, and we were already dealing with one tragedy. Four days earlier, Phil, another vice president had died of massive brain injuries resulting from a skiing accident. Operation after operation had tried to save him, each time attempting to relieve the pressure on his swollen brain, until finally, two weeks after the accident, he died. John and Phil had worked closely for years. They were both business associates and friends. John was to have given a eulogy at Phil's funeral that afternoon. Under great stress, John had written it Thursday in New York.

Art said he would take care of everything. He would find out about the medical insurance, sick leave, everything. He would tell everyone when he saw them in a couple of hours at Phil's funeral. John had so many friends, already reeling under the death of Phil. I knew they would be numb when they found out. I repeated over and over that I was so sorry this had happened. I was filled with guilt that I had not worried more.

I needed to keep telling people. Is a burden shared somehow more bearable? Does saying it make it real? My office. I needed to tell someone at my office. I owned a small training business, about fifteen employees. I called Beth, who would be in charge in my absence. Calmer, but crying, I repeated my story. She assured me that everything at work would run fine, everyone would pitch in, and she would pray for John.

Sitting on the floor teary-eyed, I saw people discreetly trying not to look at me. At that moment, I didn't care. Odd, what doesn't seem important anymore. Twenty-four hours earlier I would have been unable to imagine myself, a calm and in-control person, squatting on the floor of a hospital lobby, desperately clinging to a telephone line as if it were the umbilical cord connecting me to the real world, crying and not caring what anybody thought. I had always cared what people thought.

Enough. This had to stop. This wasn't me. If I couldn't even control myself, how could I help John? The moment passed. I took a deep breath. I stood up. I had to think. I had to plan.

Less than 45 minutes had passed. Had they started? Was John in surgery? Was he still alive? Where should I wait? Would they find me? After this, when would he be well again? What is a stroke anyway? How could I be so ignorant? When would Richard be here?

So wrapped up in my own crumbling world, I had forgotten about the rest of John's family. Where were they? Were they okay? I needed to find them.

I didn't know John's family very well. It was a second marriage for both of us. I was eleven years younger than John. His sister Kathleen and their 87 year-old mother lived together. His brother Brendan lived in Dubuque. The youngest, Mary, about my age, lived in Manhattan. I saw them mostly at weddings. John drove to Brooklyn every couple of months for an overnight visit.

When John and I married twelve years earlier, my boys were young. Visits to Brooklyn together required staying at an inconvenient hotel and left John little time to visit. He preferred going alone, sleeping on their sofa, spending more time with his family. Besides, David's and Sean's weekends were filled with baseball and soccer. John enjoyed his visits and I enjoyed the time alone with my boys. Later, after they left for college, I just enjoyed the time alone. Now I felt guilty that I didn't know John's family better because right now, I needed them.

While I was on the phone, Kathleen had gone home to see her mother, tell her what we knew, and call her brother Brendan in Dubuque. Kathleen returned. Brendan would be here as soon as possible. This morning, while we had been driving up from Maryland, someone had called John's three children. They were all coming. A call to Richard's wife confirmed that he would be arriving in a few hours.

We had garnered a row of old armless metal chairs, seats covered in green vinyl, and sat in the lobby, facing the elevator and hall, wanting to see Dr. Anant the moment he emerged from surgery. Mary to my left, Kathleen, Thomas and Jeannie to my right, we waited together, filling each other in on what we had done. This place was so public, so crowded, so filled with people waiting to see a doctor or visit a patient. Depression hung in the air. Kathleen and I, unable to sit still, walked past the room where John was in surgery, hoping but unable to see anything. We returned to the lobby. No news yet. We went to the cafeteria for coffee. Returning again, we sat in the lobby and waited. We kept reassuring each other that John was strong, that he would be okay. Why was it taking so long?

Dr. Anant appeared, still in his green surgical clothes. We sat up anxiously, stiffly on the edge of our chairs. He picked up the empty chair to Mary's left, swung it around to face us and sat down, leaning forward on his elbows. The operation was over. He spoke quietly. His voice was gentle and filled with compassion. Everything that could be done, had been done. After relaying the results of the surgery and telling us to take it one day at a time, he told us to go home. John would be in recovery for a few hours before we could see him. Then he would be moved to the neurology intensive care unit.

The news he had delivered was beginning to sink in. *If* John survived, and *if* he woke up, he could be connected to oxygen and a feeding tube, paralyzed, partially blind, unable to understand, speak, read or write, possibly with no memory, forever. It was devastating. Exhausted and teary-eyed, we got up to leave.

We were barely outside the hospital entrance when Mary uttered the most gut-wrenching, ungodly sound I had ever heard. She began to collapse and threw her arms around Kathleen, sobbing and wailing. I suddenly understood the sense of the word wailing. It came from deep within the soul, a feeling of being helpless and terrified, of tragic loss, of absolutely boundless grief. Her cries unleashed the terror we all shared. Clinging to each other for strength and comfort, we made our way to the cars.

2

The Next 48 Hours

Kathleen drove me the few blocks back to their house. John's car was parked outside. His mother was standing at the door as we arrived.

"How is he?" she asked immediately, looking distraught and as exhausted as we were. I realized guiltily that I hadn't seen her since her husband had died fifteen months earlier. She's 87 years old and her son may be dying. How difficult this must be for her.

Kathleen told her what we knew. The surgery was over. The pressure on his brain had been relieved. John was in post-op. He wouldn't wake up for at least a couple of hours. We would go back then, but we would just have to wait and see what happened. The doctor had not been very encouraging.

At 5'4" and about 130 pounds, his mother was in remarkably good health for a woman her age. But this day had taken a toll on her, as she kept reliving the events of the night before. She needed to talk and we wanted to know more about what led up to John's stroke. She told us that late Friday afternoon, John complained of a headache. He took aspirin and went upstairs to rest. Later, while she was dressing for dinner, he came back downstairs. When she returned to the living room, John was sitting on the sofa. She turned on the TV to catch the news before they left. John said he felt odd and then began pacing. He looked over at the TV.

"I can't see it right. Help me mom, something's happening." He was scared and upset.

He laid down on the sofa and kept repeating that something was wrong. Soon he couldn't stand up. He couldn't focus on the TV, then said he couldn't see it. She had been very frightened and didn't know what to do.

Fortunately, several family members live within blocks of each other in this Brooklyn community. She called Alice, her granddaughter, who lived closest. Alice's husband, Mike, answered the phone. He told her to call 911 and rushed over.

Just then her granddaughter Jeannie called to check up on her. She told Jeannie that something was wrong with John, that she had called the paramedics, but didn't know what else to do. Jeannie drove over immediately.

Minutes later Kathleen called. She told Kathleen that something was wrong with John and the paramedics were coming. Kathleen asked to speak to John.

"I can't.. I can't... I can't...," he kept repeating. Kathleen hadn't understood, thought he couldn't describe what hurt, but knew he was frightened and in pain. By the time the paramedics and Jeannie arrived, John was unable to complete a sentence. He was panicking and not making much sense. The paramedics recommended that he go to Maimonides. It was the best hospital around. His mother agreed. Jeannie went with him in the ambulance.

In retelling the story, his mom repeated several times that she hadn't known what to do. She felt guilty, as if it were her fault. We assured her over and over that she had done exactly the right thing, that no one could have done more than she did.

Why should she feel guilty, I wondered. I'm the one who should be feeling guilty. I wasn't even worrying last night. I had been annoyed that I would have to give up a weekend and drive his car back. I'm the one who deserves the guilt.

I reached my son David in Maryland by phone and told him what had happened. He was in the middle of midterms and I didn't want him leaving school. There was nothing he could do here, but he offered to call Sean in Albuquerque.

We waited for the time to pass and started to make plans. I would stay until Monday morning, drive John's car back, set things up at my office, get more clothes, and drive back on Tuesday. Now, I wanted to get back to the hospital to see John, to be there when he woke up.

I'd seen enough of those television shows where the guy wakes up, looks around, sees his family and starts talking, wanting to know where he was and what had happened. I needed to be there so I could tell him everything would be all right.

TV doesn't mirror reality. Kathleen and I were allowed to go into the recovery room. John lay still, head bandaged where the surgeon had carved open his skull, tubes in his nose, throat and arms, wires connecting his body to monitors. He hadn't awakened yet. This unreal situation kept getting more real. I felt helpless in this world where I had so little control. They asked us to leave so they could move him into the intensive care unit.

Richard arrived. I was so relieved he was there. At 6'1", with dark blonde hair, well-built and handsome, Richard was a successful attorney with a strong command presence. I welcomed his "take-charge" personality, feeling unable to do it myself. He was four years younger than I was, and though I'd never asked him for help before, I needed it now.

We went outside and sat on a park bench across the street. It was a cloudy, chilly April afternoon. Wind whipped around the tall buildings that blocked what little sun escaped the clouds. Crying again, I repeated what I had been told, wishing I understood more. How could this happen to John? It wasn't fair. He always took such good care of himself. He was in such good shape. This isn't supposed to happen to people like John.

I worried about John. Richard worried about me. I was the older sister, the self-assured bossy one, always in control of myself and my surroundings. He hadn't seen me cry in over thirty years, but now I sat beside him helpless, scared and defeated. This wasn't the sister he knew. We both needed her back.

"Who is this doctor? What do you know about him?" he asked.

"Not much. He's a neurosurgeon. He has kind eyes and a gentle, compassionate voice. He was making his rounds when the ICU doctor contacted him."

"This operation may take care of everything, but if John needs more surgery, is he the best doctor to do it? Is this the best hospital for John?"

Richard believed that if you were going to do something, you did it the best you could. If John needed more surgery, he should have the best doctor in New York, or Boston, or wherever the best doctor was.

"I don't know, Richard. I don't even know how to find out. His family seems to think this is a good hospital. I don't know anything about the hospitals in New York. I don't want to make his family angry. I don't want them to think this place is good enough for them but not good enough for us."

"You're his wife. With all due respect to his family here, you're the one who makes the decisions about John. You can't worry about hurting their feelings or making them angry. You have to do what's best for John."

"Maybe he won't need more surgery. How would I even know if another hospital is better?"

Before moving to Toronto, Richard had lived for years in New York and Boston and had contacts who might be able to help.

"I'll see what I can find out about Anant. If there's a better doctor to be taking care of John, I'll find him."

If anyone could do it, Richard could. I didn't know if we would change doctors, but I wouldn't stop Richard from checking. What I wanted was for him to discover that Dr. Anant was very competent. Over the next couple of days, he did just that. Richard's contacts in New York confirmed the doctor's good reputation. A consultation with a well-known and respected neurosurgeon affiliated with Harvard Medical School validated Dr. Anant's assessment and treatment. Dr. Anant would stay on as John's doctor.

Now in the intensive care unit, still joined by tubes and wires to machines that filled the room, John slept. Monitors beeped, and every few minutes the compression sleeves wrapped around his calves pumped up, squeezing his legs, to keep his circulation flowing. Doctors and nurses came and went. We talked quietly and watched him sleep. He opened his eyes. We jumped up in excitement, calling his name. He closed his eyes. His eyes had been open for, perhaps, two seconds. We waited. Nothing more. He slept again.

A couple of hours passed. He opened his eyes again. We reacted the same way. So did he. This time it was, maybe, five seconds. He was getting better, we assured ourselves.

Dr. Anant arrived after seven that evening. "He's woken up a couple of times," someone offered hopefully.

"How long?" he asked.

"A few seconds."

"John," he spoke loudly, trying to rouse him physically, "John, wake up."

John opened his eyes. Holding up two fingers, Dr. Anant asked loudly, "John, how many fingers do you see?" John closed his eyes. Dr. Anant examined him.

"How is he doing?" we wanted to know.

"He needs to wake up. We'll know more when he wakes up."

We asked more questions. Most of the answers were the same. It was too soon to tell. Each stroke was different. Everything was going as well as could be expected. He left. We waited some more.

John's brother Brendan had driven several hours from Dubuque to Chicago, battling an unexpected spring blizzard, to catch a plane into New York's Kennedy airport. He arrived at the hospital late that night, rushing into John's room with tears welled up in his eyes.

We updated him as John slept. We watched awhile longer, but it was getting late. Brendan asked everyone to join hands. We prayed the Lord's Prayer, then left. Richard went to a hotel. Brendan and I returned to the house with Kathleen.

A glass of white wine, an update for John's mother, a few phone calls to tell people there wasn't much to report, and we all retired. I slept soundly. It was a gift I had. When my head touched the pillow, I slept.

Early Sunday morning we returned to the hospital. Dr. Anant had already seen John and left. John had slept soundly during the night. His son, John Andrew had arrived in the early hours of the morning from Las Vegas and spent what was left of the night at Jeannie's house. John's daughter Janet and her husband Pat drove up from Maryland. His son Christopher flew in from Utah. Throughout the day, his sisters, brother, children, nieces and nephews, Richard and I, alternately took our posts, beside the bed, on the radiator, in a tiny alcove, or just holding up the walls, talking quietly among ourselves, while we waited for John to wake up.

Christopher, after questioning one of the doctors about the specific technical terminology of his father's condition, headed for the medical library to research intracerebral hemorrhages. Alternately we walked the halls, drank coffee and soda from the cafeteria, and shifted positions around the room. Someone was always by his side, holding his hand.

We watched John sleep. We waited. We worried. We left to eat. We prayed. We talked, but there didn't seem to be much to say. I couldn't think about the future. If John died—well, I couldn't think about that, and if he lived—well, I couldn't think about that either. Both alternatives seemed too horrible to contemplate. No one seemed to want to think about the future, or if they did, I wasn't privy to their thoughts.

Every couple of hours I left to go outside, to rid myself of the stifling smell. Maimonides was an old hospital. Despite the heroic efforts of the men and women who were continually scrubbing the wards, disinfectant could not completely mask the odors of age, sickness and death. The building was hermetically sealed. The odors accumulated as if they were layered, day by day, year by year with nowhere to escape. I needed to breathe fresher air, but found even outside, the smells permeated my clothes and competed with the smog in this heavily trafficked area. If John could smell it, he would have hated it too.

Mostly we waited. We were rewarded for these efforts with longer periods of wakefulness, now perhaps up to twenty seconds, every few hours. John had not spoken yet, but later in the day his eyes began to scan the room. Each time John opened his eyes, we spoke to him. Perhaps that was a smile we saw. He must recognize us. Unjustifiably optimistic, we convinced ourselves that John had seen us, that he knew we were there.

Late Sunday afternoon, Richard had to leave. He had spoken to Annie and she would be driving back up with me on Tuesday. I was so grateful that he had come.

I called John's friend Art and got the insurance information, learned that everyone had been distraught at Phil's funeral to hear about John, and that everyone was praying for his recovery.

On his evening visit, Dr. Anant roused John again, repeated the same questions, and got the same response. His examination showed no significant change, which was in itself, neither good news, nor bad news. But he had made it through the first thirty six hours.

It was Sunday night. John was still alive. He had been awake probably less than three minutes the entire day. I never thought I could spend so much time watching someone sleep. I could see why television couldn't mirror reality. For how many hours would an audience watch people watch someone sleep?

Again, with Brendan taking the lead, we joined hands, prayed the Lord's Prayer and together returned to the house.

Later that night we sat in the living room, watching the eleven o'clock news. Tiger Woods had won the Masters Golf Tournament with a spectacular 18 under par. John had been following him with interest and would have watched this game. Would he ever see Tiger Woods play again?

Feeling a terrible heavy sadness, I went out to the back porch to be alone, to cry in private. It was cold, but at least I was alone. John's daughter Janet followed and seeing me, began to cry herself. At that moment, I wanted neither to console nor to be consoled. Having been surrounded by people for two days, I needed some breathing space. I needed to grieve in private.

"Janet, I can't help you right now. You can't help me. I just need to be alone for a while. Please go back inside."

I knew I was shutting her out, but I couldn't help it. Reluctantly, she returned to the house. Brendan, hearing me cry, came outside. I wished I could have been braver, but the fear and guilt were overpowering, and the tears would not stop.

Finally, the unspeakable burst out.

"Brendan, it should have been me, not John who had the stroke. I'm the one who doesn't take care of myself. I'm the one who lives on junk food. I'm the one who hates exercise and never goes to the doctor. John does everything right. I do everything wrong. It's just not fair. It should have been me."

I'd finally said it. I'd been thinking about it for two days and I'd finally said it. If either of us deserved this, it was me, not John, but I cringed at the thought that it could have happened to me. I didn't want to die or to live the way John might be left. Even if it were possible, I couldn't asked God to spare John and take me instead. Unable to make that offer compounded my guilty and horror. I was his wife.

"Eileen, nobody wanted this to happen to John. It's crazy to think that it should have been you." He was sincere and comforting. He reached into his pocket, pulled out an immaculate white folded handkerchief, and handed it to me.

My mind took a sudden turn. Who uses handkerchiefs anymore? How many handkerchiefs had he brought with him? I would never have had a clean handkerchief at a time like this. It was ironed and folded. Did his wife iron his handkerchiefs? They must have a different kind of marriage.

"Brendan, I can't use this. I'll mess it up. It's spotless."

Now he must be certain that I had gone crazy. He laughed at me. "Go ahead, use it. Really. It's okay."

"I'll wash it before I give it back to you," I promised, embarrassed to be even using his handkerchief. I stopped. "No, I'll keep it for a while. I'll give it back when John's well." Soon I stopped crying and put it in my pocket. I felt better. Maybe my horrible thoughts weren't so horrible. Maybe each of us in our own way was feeling guilty, wondering if we should have done something different. John would get well. Brendan would get his handkerchief back another day.

It was time for bed. I had a long drive back in the morning and I was exhausted. Everyone was. Again, I slept soundly.

Monday morning, waking up early, the temporary relief I'd felt the night before was gone. I was riding on a pendulum, emotionally swinging back and forth between hope and despair. Standing in the shower, I was overwhelmed, thinking about the four hour drive back alone, my job, my career, John, my life now. What if John never knew me again? What if I spent the rest of my life taking care of a man who never knew who I was? What would be left of my life? In my mind, I saw the John I'd been staring at for two days, lying in our den, on a hospital bed, hooked up to oxygen and a feeding tube. I was sitting there holding his hand, waiting for him to wake up. Could I do this? What about me? Doesn't anybody care about me?

Suddenly filled with self-pity, I didn't think I could go on. Tears erupted again. Crumpling to the shower floor, sobbing, gasping for air, I covered my mouth, not wanting anyone to hear me. My world, my nearly perfect world, had come crashing down. I needed to hide under some covers until this nightmare ended. Despair is such a terrifying feeling. How could John do this to me?

Mary, mother of God, I prayed, please give me the strength to do whatever I have to do. Please help me. I can't do this alone. I don't know if I can do it at all. I covered my mouth and cried until I felt completely empty. Then I sat there a few minutes longer, gathering my strength until my legs could support me again.

Self-pity gave way to disgust. How could I let myself fall apart like this in someone else's house? If anyone heard me, I would be embarrassed and humiliated. Self-pity was not an emotion that was tolerated in my family. As children, whenever one of us was feeling sorry for herself, the rest of us would sit around mockingly chanting "Pity, pity, pity." We called it a pity-party. Well, I had just had mine.

"Of course you can do it," I heard what sounded like my mother's voice in my head. "You can do anything you want to do, anything you have to do." I'd heard her say it so many times before and so far, she'd always been right. I would do whatever had to be done. There was simply no other option.

"God, mom, I hope you're right," I prayed to the voices in my head. I don't know if it was an intercession from Mary, the mother of God, or from my own mother, but I do know that I felt stronger. This pity-party was over.

As I emerged from the bathroom, Kathleen asked me if I was all right. Despite the attempt to muffle my cries, the sounds had carried. Too embarrassed to admit that I had been crying for myself, and not John, I said I was fine and ended the conversation. I didn't need to publicly admit how weak and selfish I was. Better to keep this guilt private.

I called Annie to confirm that she would drive back to New York with me on Tuesday. Her husband answered. Annie had already left for work.

"Yes, she's going back up with you tomorrow. And don't worry," he added, "your father will be fine."

"My father? What's the matter with my father?"

Silence. He'd said something he wasn't supposed to say.

"Nothing," he said, trying poorly to recover.

"What's the matter with my father?" I asked louder, already anxious and very close to the edge.

"Oh, Christ, he's in the hospital, but he's going to be okay. He had a problem yesterday and they put him in the hospital, but he's okay now. He'll be coming home in a few days. I guess I wasn't supposed to tell you. Really, he's okay now," he insisted.

My family had made the decision. My plate was already full. I wasn't to be told about pop. Was this my fault? Was it because pop had learned about John's stroke? Because I'd been so upset when I called them?

I called mom immediately. She sounded calm and assured me that pop was okay. He had some bleeding in his stomach but it was under control now. He was feeling better and would be home in a couple of days. It had nothing to do with John. After hanging up the phone, I told Kathleen and her mother. Pop would be all right. I still wasn't sure it wasn't my fault, but I could only handle so much guilt and my guilt bucket was overflowing.

Time to load up the car, go see John in the hospital and drive home. I opened the front door, car keys and bags in hand. The car had been parked directly in front of the house.

"Kathleen, the car's not here. Kathleen, where's the car?" I was surprised and puzzled. Had someone moved it during the night?

Rushing to the door, Kathleen looked out. "Oh, God, it must have been stolen," she said.

"People steal cars around here?" I asked in disbelief.

"It happens. I'll call the police," she sounded irritated but calm.

How could she be so calm? It *happens*? How could she be so calm? This wasn't real. This couldn't be real. John, pop, now the car—three strikes, you're out. Torn between the choice of laughing or crying, I chose the path most traveled of late. I sat down and cried—right in front of Kathleen and her mother.

"I hate New York," I confessed, "I hate everything that's happened. I don't know what's going to happen to John. How could they steal his car?"

We all cried. It seemed to break the ice. Kathleen put her arm around me. They began to seem a little more like family.

Kathleen called the police. I called John's office. I didn't have any information about the car and needed to get the serial number and report it stolen to the insurance company. Pam, the contracting officer must be the right person.

"Pam, it's Eileen Quann. You know about John?" She did and asked how he was.

"Not good. I'll tell you about him in a minute. I know you're not going to believe this, but John's car has been stolen."

She was stunned and sympathetic, then gave me the information I needed. I updated her on John's condition and asked her to tell Art and the other people at work.

Then I called my office. My "take charge" personality was resurfacing. Beth had already told them about John. As the president of the small company, I knew that my husband's stroke affected them too and they swung into action when I told them about the car. I asked them to book me on an early afternoon flight from JFK to Baltimore. I updated them on John and before I hung up, I had my flight information. I would be in my office by late afternoon.

The police arrived. They completed their report. Kathleen and Pam together would take care of everything else regarding the car.

"Someday, we'll laugh about this day," Kathleen said.

"I hope so, but right now, it doesn't seem very funny," I responded.

As Kathleen drove me to the hospital, I thought ironically that I wouldn't have to worry about the car anymore. This was not exactly the way I would have chosen to solve the car problem. I prayed that we *would* laugh about this someday.

At Maimonides, we sat and watched John sleep for another hour. Brendan drove me to the airport. It was just past noon and it had already been a very long day.

3

The John I Knew

I was on the airplane, finally alone, allowed time for quiet contemplation. John had made it through the first 48 hours. Right or wrong, I had already ruled out the possibility that he might die. Now I wondered how he would feel about living. The John I knew was a vital person who thoroughly enjoyed life. He balanced long hours of work with travel, exercise, reading, gardening, his friends and family. He was organized and disciplined and could accomplish more in a year than most people could do in a lifetime, and he relished every minute of it. He was self-motivated, highly competitive, and liked to win, a strong type A personality. What would he be like now?

The oldest child of a very Irish, very Catholic family, John Joseph Quann was born in Brooklyn, New York on October 13, 1937. His father had emigrated from Ireland as a young man. A product of Catholic schools, John graduated from Manhattan College with a degree in Mathematics in 1959.

He immediately joined NASA at what would become Goddard Space Flight Center, working first in rented offices, then in trailers as buildings were erected around him. NASA was a new agency. The space program was the dream of a lifetime. John loved it. His career with NASA afforded opportunities and challenges that he embraced. He had a strong work ethic, a deep sense of loyalty and a belief in the value of what he was doing. He worked with engineers and scientists, both at Goddard and around the world. In his early years, he could track the trajectory of a rocket, using a slide rule, faster than the computers could. He managed projects, programs, branches, divisions and eventually rose to become the Deputy Director of Goddard Space Flight Center.

John retired from Goddard in 1988 to become a vice president of NYMA, a small company that provided engineering services for NASA and other government agencies. Over the years, he was challenged with managing and growing a business division, marketing, writing proposals, and developing strategic alliances. Would he ever work again? Would he miss it if he did not?

At 59, he had been in excellent physical condition. He planned to live to a healthy old age as his father had. What would his life be like on a feeding tube? How would he feel about being confined to a bed or a wheelchair? About having an arm that would not work?

If there is a classic charming Irishman, it was John. He loved to tell stories, and usually exaggerated. He loved a good joke. As a wedding gift to his nephew, Thomas, he offered to pay for the honeymoon—but with strings attached. Thomas and his bride would only discover at their wedding reception where they were going. Thomas was excited, his fiancee more skeptical, but they accepted his offer.

Weekly thereafter, he delighted in sending them clippings about godforsaken destinations taken from horror stories he found in travel magazines and newspapers. Bread lines behind the iron curtain, earthquakes, floods, subzero temperatures, transportation strikes, all captured his attention. At the reception, they learned their honeymoon would be in Cancun, but not before Thomas had extracted his revenge. We would discover it before the night was out.

At one in the morning the phone in our hotel room rang. "Good morning, this is your wake-up call," the cheerful recording announced. At three the phone rang, the message repeated. At five, at seven, the phone rang. "Good morning, this is your wake-up call," the recording repeated again. I was ready to kill Thomas. John loved it, thought it poetic justice. Could he still have a sense of humor when this nightmare was over?

John read a few hours every day. While he ate breakfast, he read two newspapers, skimming the headlines, occasionally reading the first paragraph, less frequently reading complete articles. At night, after dinner, he would retire into his study to pay bills, read, occasionally watch TV. He might have several books in progress at the same time, and read a little bit whenever he felt like it. John subscribed to, and read about fifteen magazines monthly, ranging from National Geographic, Sierra Club, and several travel magazines, to Biblical Archeological Review and the Jerusalem News. He read winery newsletters, and investment magazines, business and news magazines. Would he ever read again? That would be a terrible loss.

John loved to travel. He took fifteen to twenty business trips per year, plus numerous trips for pleasure, occasionally with me, sometimes with friends, often alone, frequently spontaneous. He loved to meet new people, to see new places. He was curious about everything.

John was energized by physically demanding vacations. Ten years earlier, with his children and my son Sean in tow, he rafted through the white waters of the Grand Canyon for two weeks. Two summers ago, he bicycled in Holland. He would fly to Ireland anytime for a long weekend if the fares were cheap. In fact, he would go almost anywhere for a long weekend if the fares were cheap, including Iceland in the dead of winter. On business trips to California, he stayed over the weekend to bicycle through the Napa Valley. He had organized a bicycle trip there with his sons and my brothers for next month and had signed up for another bicycle trip from Munich to Prague in July. They would need to be canceled.

Israel fascinated John so much that he flew there barely three weeks after Iraq stopped dropping scud missiles, in spite of my strenuous objections. His only concession had been to make sure his will and power of attorney were current. He had visited most of the countries in Europe, some in South America, Asia and Africa. On our cruise to Alaska, he spontaneously arranged a flight around Mount McKinley in the time it had taken me to go to the ladies' room. Last January, we spent three weeks in Australia and New Zealand. We both enjoyed the snorkeling, hiking, horseback riding, and white water rafting. John parasailed off the side of a mountain while my fear of heights and love of shopping kept my feet planted firmly on the ground in the local shops. I reluctantly acquiesced to his insistence that I join him on the early morning black water rafting trip. After donning icy wet suits and head lamps, we alternately trudged through caves rippling with icy glacier water and live eels, and floated on inner tubes as the cave expanded, ultimately to fall backwards over a rushing waterfall into a black pit an unseen distance below. For three long hours, as I listened to the distant echo of the rushing waters ahead, he was exuberant while I was terrified.

He had spoken to me recently about taking time off from work to travel, gradually easing into retirement. I was 48 years old, with many more "working" years ahead of me. Several of the places John yearned to see didn't interest me. We had thought that three or four extended trips a year for a few years should get it out of his system. Would he travel again?

John found pleasure in working in the yard. He loved spring because he could start planting again. He anticipated the arrival of his hummingbirds every summer and the Canadian geese in the fall. This man even liked mowing the lawn.

Though a light drinker, he enjoyed microbrewery beers and good wine. Somehow, he managed to find a microbrewery in every city we visited. He would often bring a new wine or beer back for a friend. They would do the same for him.

Time for a reality check. John had a lot of virtues, but he was no saint. The man I married could be critical, impatient and quick to anger. He was stubborn, proud and judgmental. He was incapable of saying either "I'm sorry" or "I was wrong" and we could go for days without speaking after a fight. He was fiercely competitive, often even with me, and our marriage was an odd struggle between being highly supportive and highly critical, both with equal amounts of enthusiasm.

We had both changed a lot since I met John when he was the deputy director at Goddard, but I had fond memories of our beginning. In September 1982, I was a contractor managing a team of software developers at Goddard. I had been separated for fifteen months and was raising my five and six year old sons alone. Their father, an army officer, had gone to Germany on a three year assignment when we separated. It was a Friday afternoon and the center was replacing a huge, old computer. I was attending "The Death of the IBM 360 Party" before I had to leave work to pick up my kids. I had had a glass of wine, unusual for me that time of day since I rarely took time for breakfast or lunch, and it put me in a cocky mood.

I turned to Mike, my boss's boss and said, "Point me in the direction of a single man."

Just then, John walked into the room. Mike, hearing the challenge in my voice, pointed to John, as if daring me to make a move.

"Isn't that the deputy director?" I asked.

He nodded.

"Are you absolutely sure he's single?"

Again he nodded.

"You'd better be right or...," my voice trailed off, deciding against a threat.

"What's the matter, are you afraid?" he taunted.

That did it. Bravely I walked over and started up a conversation. For the next thirty minutes, we must have talked, although I can't remember a thing that was said. I knew if John wanted to leave, he would, but as long as Mike was watching, I wasn't going anywhere. The wine ran out, there hadn't been that much. People were leaving. John asked me if I'd like to go to Jasper's, a popular bar, and have a drink. This was definitely not the time to tell him I had two small children who had to be picked up at day care in less than an hour. Trying to be calm and casual, as if this were an everyday event, I said I'd like that, but had to check on something first. Excited and frantic, I ran to the phone. Annie, please be home. She answered, thank God. My voice bubbled over.

"Annie, I need a really, really big favor. You're not going to believe this! This guy, actually, he's the deputy director of Goddard, just asked me to go have a drink with him. I need for you to pick up Sean at Montessori school by five thirty and David at after-school by six. I promise I'll do anything in the world for you if you'll do this, just please say yes. I shouldn't be more than two hours. Please, please, can you do it?"

Annie agreed, assuring me that I would owe her big time. I returned to John looking calm. We went for a drink. He was charming, but one drink was my limit. Unlike Cinderella, I was watching the clock. He walked me to my car and said he'd call. I said I'd like that.

No call.

A month later, I saw him at another function. We chatted for a few minutes. He said he'd call.

No call.

A couple of weeks later, I sent him a birthday card. No response. Why do men say they'll call when they have no intention of calling? I gave up.

Early December, three months later, the phone rang.

"Hi, this is John Quann."

"John Quann?" stalling, I needed a second to control the excitement in my voice. He was actually calling!

"Yeah, remember me? I told you I'd call."

"Yes, but so soon!" I replied, reluctant to forgive him so quickly, reaching for sarcasm to cover my excitement.

And so the relationship began. John was handsome, smart and funny, generous and sexy. He took me to exciting places, to dances and formal functions. I was swept away by his Irish charm. He was important, and I was impressed, and somewhat intimidated by his position.

Three months into the relationship, John made it clear that he had no intention of remarrying. The romantic in me believed he would fall in love, decide he couldn't live without me, and change his mind. A year and a half later, I had accepted the fact that John was not the marrying kind but I believed that my boys needed a father. I didn't want them growing up believing that men could have the fun part of marriage without the responsibilities. Another man had asked me out. My relationship with John seemed to be going nowhere. Regretfully, I believed it was over and told John I was accepting the invitation. John called two days later and asked me to marry him. Less than a year after that, we marched down the aisle.

Ours wasn't an easy marriage. I came to believe in later years that it was mostly my fault, not because John was blameless, but because I, not John, was the one who had changed. My self-esteem had been badly damaged by the failure of my first marriage, and in the beginning, I didn't think I deserved someone as wonderful as John. He controlled the relationship, and I let him, anxious to please and impress him. As I healed and became stronger, I resented what I perceived as the one-sidedness of it all. I argued that I didn't want to control John, I just didn't want him to control me either. From my perspective, fights were almost always, somehow, over his need to control me. Suddenly now I wondered, did John now have complete control over me, dragging me into his hellish prison, or I over him, making every decision for him? Either way, I didn't see how it could be good.

We spent most of our married years struggling to carve out the space in which our marriage could work. At times it seemed impossible. To survive together, we began to distance ourselves from each other. The years when David and Sean were teenagers were particularly difficult. Suffice it to say, he thought I was too lenient. I thought he was unreasonable. Childrearing was a challenge we almost didn't survive.

Before our marriage, we had each spent years as single parents and had established ourselves professionally. To both of us, freedom and independence were valued and expected rights. We each traveled frequently on business and neither resented it.

Once, at a party, John was discussing a trip he had made that week. Standing a few feet away and overhearing him mention the airport in Atlanta, I interrupted.

"John, when were you in the Atlanta airport?"

"Thursday night."

"What time?"

"Between six and eight."

"What airline?"

"Delta."

"What gate?"

"I don't know, 17, I think. Why?

"John, I was at gate 19 then. I was coming from Montgomery to Baltimore. What were you doing there?"

"I had a meeting in Birmingham that afternoon and was going through Atlanta to Orlando."

Our friends witnessing this conversation were astonished. I was amazed at the coincidence. The incident was a reminder of how extensively we both traveled, and of how separate our lives often were.

Winters were the most stressful season. I hated cold weather and commuting in the dark. I hated feeling cooped up. Since my homicidal instincts were stronger than my suicidal ones, John took the brunt of my weather-induced hostility. But he wasn't much better. By late February of every year he was ready to move out, and I was ready to help him pack. It was only in the last couple of years that we saw the pattern and realized that sunshine and warm weather were critical to our relationship. It was then that we began taking winter vacations to warmer, sunny climates and life improved.

In fact, it seemed that only in the past year had we finally been able to reach an accommodation. In our unwritten, unspoken arrangement, I knew we shared respect for both our professional and personal lives, mutual trust, and admiration for our successes. We were both genuinely interested in each other's careers and most conversations revolved around work. We enjoyed vacationing and dining out together. With my boys away at college, the stress of parenting had diminished. We had defined the boundaries of what we were willing to share.

Love wasn't a word either of us felt comfortable with, nor one we would have used to characterize our relationship. Neither of us was sentimental, and friends laughed at us because neither of us knew the date or year we were married. If we needed to know for some reason, we'd call his mother and ask. She remembered such details. Otherwise, we celebrated the last Saturday in June if we remembered that much, or maybe we'd go out to dinner in July and call it our anniversary if we forgot. Maybe not. It wasn't that big a deal.

John wasn't physically demonstrative and would accept, but never initiate, a hug, or holding hands. It was something I needed and missed, but had come to accept. It sometimes surprised me that we slept so perfectly together. Sex and affection were separate, compartmentalized activities. Would there ever be any physical side to our relationship again?

We both had full lives outside our marriage, and I thought we were content. We gave each other a lot of space. Now, suddenly, unexpectedly and unfairly, the rules had changed.

Could John survive if he were totally dependent on me, or anybody else? Would he resent my being able to do things that he could not do himself? Would he come to hate me? Could I survive it? Would we both become prisoners of his stroke?

As much as I wondered if the gifts John had would be lost, I feared all the negatives could be reinforced. We hadn't always thought we could survive together before. Could our marriage survive this? If it couldn't, what could I do? And what would happen to John?

The plane was landing in Baltimore. Perhaps the time alone for quiet contemplation hadn't been such a good idea. I certainly didn't feel any better and dreaded what lay ahead.

4

Alone at Home

I caught a cab home, mentally planning what I needed to do before returning to New York the next day. Dr. Anant had said that John would only be at Maimonides for a couple of weeks. I needed to find another place for John, either a nursing home or a rehabilitation facility. Coming home was not an option. I had no experience dealing with serious illness. I jumped in panic for a nurse every time a monitor beeped. Beyond holding his hand or rubbing his arm, I was almost afraid to touch him, afraid of hurting him. I was uncomfortable with the intimate nature of the caregiver role, embarrassed by the thought of cleaning him when he relieved himself. Someday I might have to do it but there was no way I could take care of him now. He needed a lot more help than I was able give him, but a nursing home wasn't acceptable to me either. Those were ending places, not starting places. I had to believe that John was going to get well. I needed to find a place where he could.

I also needed to find out more about our insurance—to know what was covered by our plan. I still had a business to run, but it would survive without me for a couple of weeks. This was the best month the company had ever had. I could count on the people at the office to manage with minimal oversight until I found a longer-term solution.

I needed to learn more about strokes. Our lives had taken a horrible unexpected turn and I didn't understand enough about what was happening to John. I had to believe he could recover, but I had no idea how much recovery we could expect. I wanted to spend as much time with him as I could, to help him however I could. Angry with myself for being so ignorant, I was determined to learn more.

Once before my life had been in emotional turmoil. In the early months of being a single parent, I operated in what I called survival mode, where I established a very limited set of priorities, delegated what I could, and ignored everything else. For the second time in my life, I would function in survival mode until I could manage more.

My first call was to the insurance company. First calls—to be exact. After several wrong numbers, each containing a long series of "if you want...push 1, if you need...push 2," I finally made contact with a human being by pretending to be on a rotary phone and just staying on the line. Not the right human being of course, but someone who could tell me how to contact the right human being. After that, it was almost easy. Almost. This was the first time I had to tell a stranger what had happened. My emotions were still too raw to relay the events of the last three days without crying. With difficulty, I explained what had happened and found myself talking to an understanding and helpful person.

He told me what I needed to do, what they would do, what our insurance covered, and for how long. I told him that John would need to go someplace else in a couple of weeks. He said that we should have a book that listed all the facilities in our plan.

He answered other questions and said that John would have a caseworker assigned to his case. He gave me his direct line and told me to call if I had any other questions. Before leaving for New York the next day, John's caseworker had contacted me. She gave me her direct phone number and told me to call if I had any questions or problems.

I was amazed and relieved by the support they provided. Though I'd had little contact with insurance companies in the past, I didn't remember ever hearing anything good about them, especially when you needed them. I had expected detached voices that would recite the rules and tell me all the limitations, and discovered instead caring human beings.

The book that listed rehabilitation facilities was filed in John's desk in a folder marked "Medical Insurance". Thank God John was so organized. There were several facilities listed in Maryland, Virginia and DC, but I had no idea which ones might be appropriate, or would accept him. How in the world does one as ignorant as I go about screening rehabilitation facilities? I planned to spend some time on the Internet, to see what services they offered, to narrow my search before calling them. I was only home for a few hours and there was still much to do. I'd be home again on Thursday and should know a lot more about John's condition then. On to the next task.

Needing someone to pick up the newspapers and mail, I walked next door. Carol, our neighbor, was home. I blurted out what had happened to John. Her kindness and concern opened the floodgates behind my eyes. I felt so embarrassed to be crying. Usually I'm objective, somewhat detached. Now I was fragile, vulnerable to kindness. I felt like a soft-shell crab, stripped of my protective covering by the shock of John's stroke, my insides exposed and unbearably sensitive. The gentlest touch, the smallest kindness, or show of sympathy, sent ripples of pain through my body and tears to my eyes.

Together we cried and hugged. She wanted to help. She agreed to take care of the mail and newspapers. She knew someone who lived nearby whose husband had a stroke a couple of years ago and offered to introduce us. I told her I'd be back on Thursday and would like to meet her friend then if possible.

A quick call to Annie confirmed that we would leave about nine the following morning.

"It's a good thing you want me to go with you," she said.

"Why's that?"

"Because Richard called and said, 'No matter what she tells you, go with her.'" She laughed. It was my first smile in three days. We hung up. My family doesn't think I have it all together yet, I realized. Thank God for family.

At the office, I was greeted with stricken, sympathetic looks and subdued voices. Calling everyone into the conference room, I updated them on John's condition. I explained that I would be dividing my time between New York and home for the next couple of weeks. They already knew John's car had been stolen and I told them I wasn't anxious to take my new Chrysler Sebring convertible up to Brooklyn, but didn't have much choice. Someone recommended "The Club", a device that locks onto a car's steering wheel. Such security precautions were foreign to me, but I wrote it down.

They would have to run the office. I trusted them to make any decisions that had to be made. They assured me that everything would be fine and all offered to pray for John. I delegated work, signed checks, answered questions and promised to stop back on Thursday.

It was five o'clock. Alone with the whole night ahead of me, the first stop was Trac Auto to purchase "The Club". Expecting I'd have to explain it to him, I was surprised when the man behind the counter knew immediately what I wanted, and I was reminded again of my own naiveté.

Next stop, the bookstore. Borders was huge, and though I'd been there many times, my knowledge of the health section was limited to the latest diet books. I was afraid to ask someone if they had any books on strokes. I was afraid I would cry. Eventually, I found *Family Guide to Stroke*, published by the American Heart Association, which looked like my best bet. It was in English, not technical jargon. It described the different kinds of strokes, the surgery John had, rehabilitation and living with a disabled person.

Disabled—that word had a jarring sound. We weren't the kind of people who had the word disabled associated with them. That label was for other people, people your mother taught you to be kind to, people you taught your children not to stare at. Not people we knew, not John. Suddenly I hated labels. Averting my eyes, I paid the cashier, afraid I would see a questioning or sympathetic look, paranoid that I would feel compelled to explain why I was buying it, afraid I would cry.

Returning home, I called David and Sean. There was no point in their coming home. It was near midterms and there wasn't anything they could do here. Watching John sleep wasn't an option for them. I had already spoken to them from New York and there was little new to report.

The doorbell rang. It was Rick, a new neighbor I had met a couple of times, briefly. Working at Goddard himself, he had learned of John's stroke in a staff meeting that morning. Word travels fast. Everyone at Goddard must know by now. Relieved at having that task taken from me, I wondered how they found out. Art or someone at Phil's funeral must have told them.

"How's John doing?" Rick asked.

"Well, he's survived the surgery and the first forty-eight hours. That's the good news. He's in intensive care, hooked up to all sorts of machines. Mostly, he's sleeping. The doctors aren't very encouraging. They expect him to be paralyzed. They don't know whether he'll be able to speak, or read or write or understand us. It's too soon to know much." I could feel the pressure of water behind my eyes, the thickness in my throat. I didn't want to cry.

"Listen," he said kindly, rescuing me from a tearful display, "last fall I bought a new riding lawnmower. It was so late in the season, I hardly got a chance to use it. I was wondering if you'd mind if I mowed your lawn when I mow mine."

"Would I mind?" I felt my second smile in as many hours. "You make it sound like I'm doing you a favor. No, Rick, I wouldn't mind. It would help me a lot. I wasn't sure how I was going to take care of the lawn right now. Thank you so much."

He promised to mow it in a couple of days and left. That was one acre less to worry about. Thank you Rick. Thank you Lord for my kind neighbors.

A call to John's mother in Brooklyn revealed that Kathleen was at the hospital and John was still sleeping most of the time. She promised to call if there was any change. I would be back up in the morning.

Not hungry, I sat down in my favorite recliner and opened the book *Family Guide to Stroke*. There was so much to learn.

John had had an intracerebral hemorrhage. This occurs when an artery deep within the brain ruptures and blood flooding into the brain tissue destroys it. Only about ten percent of all strokes were of this type. Intracerebral hemorrhages were not only the least common type of stroke, they also had the poorest survival rate—only about ten percent of victims survived, and John's had been severe.

The most common culprit is high blood pressure, but that had not been John's problem. Dr. Anant suspected that the cause was an AVM, an arteriovenous malformation, but it had not been confirmed with an angiogram.

This can occur when a thick-walled artery is connected to a thin-walled vein, a birth defect of sorts. When blood pressure shoots up, the connection can burst. Perhaps it was only because John always had low blood pressure and excellent health that he had never had a problem before. Had the stroke been triggered by Phil's death, or by recent stress at the office? We'd probably never know.

John had none of the risk factors for stroke. Always a sucker for those self-tests, I filled out the stroke risk profile. John scored only 2 points out of a possible 30, putting him in the 3% risk category and that was only because he was over 50. A little late to be relieved—statistics obviously don't tell the whole story, and they sure don't mean much when it happens to you. The kind of stroke John had, if it was caused by an AVM, wasn't addressed by these risk factors.

I highlighted paragraphs as I read, searching for those sections most relevant to John's condition.

Hematomas can cause periods of unconsciousness. Patients with very large hematomas over their dominant cerebral hemisphere have a smaller chance of recovery. For them, neither surgery nor medication is likely to be of much help.

I was beginning to understand why the doctor was so guarded in his prognosis for John. The book went on to list all the complications of stroke: edema, often following a brain hemorrhage, when the brain swells, causing further brain damage; heart problems; blood vessel problems; bed sores; limb contractures, where the paralyzed side of the body "freezes" in position; arthritis; pneumonia; seizures; depression.

I needed to know these things, and torn between hating what I was learning, and not being able to put the book down, I continued reading.

The chapter on rehabilitation gave me ideas about what I needed to look for in a facility. It was there that I learned the difference between physical therapy which addresses the lower body, and occupational therapy which addresses the upper body. Speech therapy involved much more than speech. It was concerned with a patient's ability to understand what was said, to speak, read, write and even swallow. From what I was reading, his prognosis was not good for any of these problems. The only things John seemed to have going for him were his excellent health and high intelligence before the stroke and his relatively young age. Motivation to recover was also critical, but it was too soon to determine that.

Our house, I realized in the next chapter, was very inaccessible to someone in a wheelchair, assuming John would even be able to use one. In spite of its contemporary looking cedar-sided exterior and high slanted roofs, our home was basically a two story, four bedroom, two and a half bath colonial with an attached sunroom. Whether one entered through the front door, the two car garage or any of the three sliding glass doors off the multi-level deck, there were stairs to navigate, and inside, the hall stairway had a 90° turn. The bathroom doorways were too narrow for wheelchair passage. There was no full bath downstairs. Would I have to convert the downstairs sunroom into a bedroom and add a full bathroom? There was even a step down from the living room into the sunroom, and heating and central air barely reached it, leaving the sunroom too warm in the summer and too cold in the winter.

John's son Christopher worked as an architect in Salt Lake City, specializing in hospital renovations, but I didn't know an architect in this area. How much would it cost? We loved this house. Would John ever be able to live here again? Would I have to sell it? Would I need to find an apartment temporarily when John came home? Those problems were simply too overwhelming to worry about now.

I read into the early hours of the morning. As I reached the final chapter, it was beginning to sink in how long this journey might be. I had obtained some information, but not much hope and I had barely scratched the surface. There was still a lot more reading to do. Three days ago, John was functioning at one hundred percent. Today, lying in his hospital bed in the intensive care unit, John was alive. He had gone from a hundred percent to nearly zero in a matter of hours. Exhausted again, I went to bed.

$\approx$ 5 $\approx$

Inch Pebbles of Progress

Sleeping soundly didn't guarantee that I would wake up feeling rested, but I was anxious to see John again. After packing a few things and throwing "The Club" in the back seat, I picked up Annie. The drive was uneventful until, as we approached New York, Annie struggled to rip off the heavy stiff plastic encasing the club, trying to avoid cutting her hands on the sharp edges in the process. We considered stopping to buy a blow torch, but rejected the idea—too time consuming. Besides, neither of us knew how to operate one. We speculated about whether we could just buy the plastic and wrap the car in it. No one would be able to steal it then. Amused but defeated, the still packaged club was returned to the back seat.

It was almost noon. Around the hospital, cars were double-parked. The hospital parking lot was full, but I pulled in behind two other cars that were waiting. A young man approached.

"You can't park here," he told me.

"I have to. My husband's had a stroke. We just drove up from Maryland. I don't know where else to go." I was ready to beg if I had to. Parking in New York was not something I was prepared to cope with now, especially after John's car had been stolen just yesterday. Was it only yesterday? My life was beginning to feel like a video, alternating between slow motion and fast forward.

"How long will you be here?" he asked.

Was he more likely to take my car if I said a few minutes or a few hours? I'd try honesty first. If that didn't work, then maybe I'd beg. Crying wouldn't have been difficult either.

"Until dinner time," I responded hopefully.

"Leave the car here and give me your keys," he said.

I thanked him profusely. Annie and I jumped out of the car before he could change his mind.

Entering the ICU, I found John sleeping, his son John Andrew holding his hand. John Andrew had spent years valet parking cars in Las Vegas. I told him about the man who so graciously took my car, and about the Club, now encased in torn, ironclad plastic, laying in the back seat.

"Was he wearing a uniform?" he asked.

"I don't think so."

"Do you have the keys to the car?"

"No, he took them."

"Did he give you a ticket?" he asked hopefully.

"No," I said more slowly, as my good Samaritan in the parking garage began to sprout horns.

"You handed your car keys over to a man who wasn't wearing a uniform, left the car with him, told him you'd be gone for hours, didn't get a ticket, and left the club in the back seat of your car?" he repeated, looking at me as though I'd just been had.

"Yes," I confessed as the thought of a second stolen car in two days began to take shape.

"Why don't we just go down and check?" he suggested.

John Andrew and I walked to the parking lot and approached the attendant in the booth. The man didn't know anything about the car. Just as panic was beginning to set in, the familiar young man appeared. Yes, he had parked the car. Yes, it was over there, he said grinning, pointing to the car in an alley across the street. I was embarrassed that I had thought the worst, and relieved that I still had a car.

John Andrew gave him a generous tip and told him that I would be spending a lot of time at the hospital in the next couple of weeks. John retrieved the car keys, somehow removed the club from the casing and showed me how to work it. After that, they remembered me, and I always had a parking space. I often left it there overnight, afraid to park on the street where John's car had been stolen. When, after long days and nights at the hospital, I forgot where it was parked, they even told me. The men at the parking garage treated me well.

John's periods of wakefulness were increasing. His left arm, which he could still use, now had to be strapped to the bed railing unless someone sat beside him, holding his hand. During the night, he had ripped out the naso-gastric tube that went through his nose and into his stomach to feed him. Replacing it was a major undertaking, requiring that X-rays be taken, developed and read to make certain the tube was properly inserted into his stomach before the equipment could be hooked up again. As a result, hours elapsed while John had no nutrition.

It was obvious that he didn't like the tubes in his nose and mouth. He continually tried to reach for them, to pull them out. Did explaining it to him make any difference? We tried, but I kept wondering if he knew what was going on. He had not spoken, had not responded to any of us yet, had done nothing beyond briefly opening his eyes and looking around his room. Could he understand that he needed those tubes? Selfishly, I wanted him to know what was happening, to know I was here for him. On the other hand, I doubted that I would have wanted to know any of this, if I were John.

By Tuesday night, he no longer needed oxygen—our first big breakthrough. John's breathing would be okay! Images of an oxygen tank in our den for the rest of his life evaporated. He was getting better. There was still no movement in his right arm or leg. He was still unable to respond when Dr. Anant, twice each day, held up two fingers and asked him how many fingers he saw, but he could breathe without equipment. I believed the tide was turning.

By Wednesday, a machine with a hydraulic lift moved him from the bed to a chair for a couple of hours to reduce the possibility of bedsores. He was awake longer now. He seemed more aware of what was going on around him. He smiled. He was never without family, except in the middle of the night. Usually there were a few people, someone always holding his hand. If John was awake when a new person entered the room, he reached out for them, as if he needed to feel human contact. He touched everyone. He held on to everyone.

I marveled at this. It was so unlike John. Is the touch of another human being the most primitive form of contact? Did he need to feel someone to know that he was alive?

He had begun to utter a few words. His vocabulary now included "yes, no, listen, stop, wow, oh my goodness, and thank you." The doctor called this automatic speech, words that are spoken automatically, without thought, over which there is little control. He explained that this didn't mean John could understand us, or could use meaningful speech. At one point, waking up to see several of us watching him, he said, "I am so, so sorry." That was his only meaningful sentence for a while. He knew something had happened to him. We tried to explain, but he didn't seem to understand. Was it like waking up in a foreign land, where nobody spoke your language?

There had still been no movement in his right arm or leg, despite our efforts to work them following the instruction of the hospital staff. The doctor was discouraging. It didn't look like John would get any movement back in his right side.

Annie and I returned home Thursday afternoon. She stayed when my neighbor Carol and her friend arrived to talk about rehabilitation facilities. Carol's friend described her husband, a young man, who had a severe stroke two years earlier. She talked about his condition and the extent of his recovery. He had returned to work, but was still significantly impaired. He never fully recovered physically and walked, using a cane, with great difficulty. He had gone to Sinai in Baltimore following his stroke. She also recommended Kernan Rehabilitation Facility, affiliated with the University of Maryland Medical System, which was closer and had opened a new wing with a stroke unit after her husband's stroke. She brought business cards of people at both places.

Later that evening I located Kernan on the Internet. The facility was new and modern. It offered physical, occupational and speech therapy in a special unit for stroke survivors, but I wasn't sure John was ready for it. He had only been off oxygen for one day, and was still on a feeding tube. He slept most of the day, wasn't communicating, and had no sensation in his right arm or leg. They might not even take him, but I only had a week to find a place. Did rehabilitation facilities have waiting lists?

Friday I called Kernan. I spoke to a woman who suggested that we meet on Tuesday, the next time I would be back in Maryland. That was cutting it close. What if it wasn't the right place, or they couldn't take him?

I stopped by the office for a couple of hours, then drove to the library. The librarian helped me find several articles and books, including one written by a man who had had a stroke years before. Friday night I read everything I had. The technical information was difficult to understand. Because intracerebral hemorrhages are uncommon and survival rare, I didn't find much literature on recovery statistics. The book written by the stroke survivor offered hope for John's recovery, but it had taken years of hard work before he could speak, read or write. The author had spent his first six months in denial and depression. Less than a week had passed and I was exhausted. I'd never make it through years of this. How would John and I ever survive? Discouraged again, well past midnight, I went to bed.

Saturday my brother Paul arrived from Houston. He had a meeting in New Jersey on Monday and would drive with me to Brooklyn. My family was watching out for me and I was grateful. Remembering John's love of music, Paul bought a boom box and some CDs that John could listen to in the hospital.

We arrived at Maimonides Saturday afternoon. John was awake and reached out with his left hand to touch me. He tried to get his fingers underneath the cuff of my long sleeve shirt. As I unbuttoned it, he stroked my arm, seeking the contact, the connection. Surely he must know who I am. He does know who I am, doesn't he? John no longer had a feeding tube. That morning he had "passed" the swallowing test and would now be able to eat solid food. Another leap forward. Images of John connected to a feeding tube at home evaporated. Thank you God, he's getting better.

Though he still slept most of the day, he was awake now for up to thirty minutes at a time, and was moved into a chair for several hours each day. He had a constant stream of visitors. He seemed to recognize people, and each of us believed he knew who we were. He smiled at each new visitor, laughed when we laughed, and seemed to be listening when we spoke to him. John still couldn't respond when Dr. Anant held up two fingers and asked him how may fingers he saw. He simply looked puzzled. Did he understand what anyone said to him or was he only responding to our body language?

Early that evening, when Dr. Anant made his rounds, John's right foot responded with the tiniest movement to Dr. Anant's prodding. We were all elated. One week had elapsed since his surgery. The doctor took me out into the hallway and made his first promising prediction.

"It looks like John may walk again, though he will probably need a walker or platform cane. He has some sensation in his foot, and that's a good sign. He will need a lot of physical therapy, but he will probably walk again."

"What about his arm?" I asked, daring to hope for more.

"That doesn't look very good. He still has no sensation or movement. His arm will probably curl up, and may lock in this position." He held his right arm at his side, elbow and wrist bent, fingers awkwardly curled up on his chest, demonstrating what I could expect. As a child, I had a great aunt with arthritis whose arm looked like that. John would hate that.

Torn between the relief of John being mobile in the future and the dismal prognosis for his arm, I decided to concentrate on the mobility. The arm might come back later. For now, we'd focus on the positive.

By Saturday night, it looked like John had escaped death, and was on the road to recovery. He was awake, smiling and had a room full of visitors to celebrate. There were thirteen people, to be exact, crowded into his tiny ICU room. Paul and I were there. His sisters, children, nieces and nephews, had come to cheer him up. The doctors had warned us that his memory might be faulty, and his nieces and nephews were speculating on whether he would remember the stories he had told over the years at their expense. That night, the younger generation decided to set the record straight, to reconstruct his stories, this time telling their versions, jokingly suggesting that John would remember only the version he heard that night.

The most famous was the summer beach story when the kids were young and "uncle" John had taken them to Dairy Queen, telling them to order anything they wanted. In the version John had told for years, young Thomas had ordered a banana split, telling the waitress to hold the whipped cream, nuts, topping and bananas. John had paid for a banana split; Thomas was eating a dish of vanilla ice cream! John had gone crazy. Thomas, the tough New York cop, in his thick Brooklyn accent, retold the story, claiming that only the nuts had been omitted, that he had been given a "bum rap". We were all laughing, suspecting the truth was somewhere in between.

The sign at the entrance to the ICU limited visitors to two at a time, but so far, the doctors and nurses had been very tolerant and we had been quiet and well behaved. We were pushing our luck that night when the head doctor walked past and looked quite startled to see what could only have been described as a party going on. This was a strict Hassidic Jewish hospital. We were breaking all their rules.

I rushed out to meet him, torn between panic and contrition, but still laughing over Thomas's infamous banana split. Anticipating his reaction to the number of people in the room, I looked him straight in the eye.

"Doctor, they're Irish. They can't count."

His frown almost turned into a smile.

Trying to placate him, I volunteered, "John looks good, doesn't he? He's really enjoying this. And everyone is so relieved. And, um, several of them will be leaving soon."

"Keep the noise down, or they'll be leaving *very* soon."

"Thank you, we will," I promised. John dozed off soon afterwards and we all left.

During John's stay at Maimonides, I got to know his mother and sister much better. His mother, at 87 years old, still had a sharp mind, a traditional Irish Catholic devotion to God, and a great kindness about her. On the occasions she sat beside his bed, holding his hand, she prayed with her rosary.

A love of reading ran in the family. Though her eyesight was poor, John's mom still read for a good part of the day, using both strong reading glasses and a magnifying glass, reading slowly, one word at a time, as she passed the magnifying glass over the large print. She was warm and kind to me and I began to call her mom. It was easier and felt comfortable.

Kathleen was always there—for John, for me, for her mother and her family. She continued to work, cutting back her hours. She would arrive at the hospital early in the morning, stay as long as she could before commuting to the office, and then return after work. She scheduled time off to be at the hospital when I was in Maryland, and went into the office on the days I was at the hospital. I was amazed by her organizational skills and her energy, and grateful for her support.

Both John's and my families were very supportive. In the moments when I could distance myself from it, I was fascinated by the different role each person played. Everyone was clearly concerned and involved. There was no conscious master plan at work, yet each person found a unique way to contribute. The crisis showed a side of each person that I had not fully appreciated before and the diversity intrigued me.

Christopher spent hours in the medical library, learning about his father's stroke, sharing what he learned every day with the rest of us. Alice, Kathleen's oldest daughter, prepared delicious meals (her eggplant parmesan my favorite) and brought them over to mom's house at night. Mary was there with emotional support, holding my hand, hugging me, taking notes. Steve, her husband, searched the Internet for information on rehabilitation facilities. Brendan, with his strong shoulder and clean handkerchiefs, saw his share of my tears, and with his wife Jeanne back in Dubuque, prayed for John. Janet, torn between sick children at home in Maryland and her father in the hospital in New York, drove back and forth several times. She was the optimist, always looking for the tiniest signs of improvement, constantly trying to cheer us up.

Kathleen opened her home to me and my family, filling every need, often before it was voiced. Thomas, dropping in every day, even if only for a few minutes at lunch, was quick with the joke to make everyone laugh. Richard, as a brother was emotionally supportive. As a lawyer, he researched Dr. Anant, wanting to find the best doctor for John. Paul brought music and companionship. Annie was there for me, day or night, never more than a phone call away, to spend the night, or talk, or just listen. David and Sean called often, checking to see how both John and I were doing. My neighbors took in the mail and papers, mowed the lawn and watched over the house. And John Andrew, bless his soul, sat beside his father for hours at a time, holding his hand, rubbing his arm, speaking quietly to him, telling him he would be all right, that he would get better. I was not alone in this, and though there were moments when alone held tremendous appeal, I knew how lucky John and I were.

Slowly we watched John progress. In business, we measured progress in milestones. I was reminded of a phrase I once heard that described an enormous task in which progress was painstakingly slow. At Maimonides, we could measure his improvement in "inch pebbles".

6

Taking Charge

I had transitioned from the initial shock and raw emotions of the first forty-eight hours, dependent on those around me, into full gear. Now, it seemed, I was busy every minute. I was in contact with many of John's friends from Goddard and NYMA through e-mail and the phone, keeping them abreast of his condition. I worked several hours at the office on the days that I was home. Alone at night, I was reading, learning about strokes and rehabilitation, searching for the next stop for John. I spoke with caseworkers almost daily, keeping them informed, asking questions, getting help. I updated at least one member of my family every day, trusting them to spread the word. I spent every moment I could with John. The car and the hospital became my new temporary homes. Keeping busy helped, there was no time for tears. There were more important things to do.

Sunday, after I left for Maryland, John was moved out of the ICU. His vital signs were stable and he no longer needed to be connected to equipment that monitored him. His home for the next few days was called a step-down unit, one level of care below the ICU. It was a large room with four occupied beds and a nurse's station in the center.

When I returned Monday afternoon, and entered his room, the nurse quickly informed me that only family was allowed. Surprised, I told her that I was his wife. She had assumed Kathleen was since Kathleen had been there when he was moved. It was a logical assumption. My initial irritation at having my place usurped was replaced with wry humor.

"I know married couples grow to look like each other, but brothers and sisters start off that way."

We laughed. John might not know I was his wife, but at least now his nurse did.

John looked better just sleeping in a regular hospital bed. Because he was now sharing a room with three other patients, the nurses strictly enforced the two-visitor limit and insisted on rest times when no visitors were allowed. Family members now found themselves spending more time in the tiny waiting area than visiting with John. His kids needed to get back to their jobs. Things began to quiet down.

When I arrived Tuesday morning, he was awake and sitting in a chair. His breakfast tray had arrived—orange juice, yogurt, cereal, Jell-O and coffee. Until now, family members, wanting to help, had fed him. I was a big believer in helping people to be independent. As a single parent, it was a necessary act of survival. By the time my youngest was four years old, they both made their own breakfasts, Sean climbing up onto the counter to microwave his oatmeal every morning, David pouring the milk for him when the gallon jug was full. When David was seven and foolishly complained that his soccer shirt and socks had not been cleaned, they were taught how to operate a washing machine. After that, they did their own laundry. I was more willing to discover that an entire load consisted of two socks and a shirt than I was to resume the chore myself. I believed the fastest way for John to recover was to encourage him do as much as he could for himself. And finally, for the first time in ten days, I was alone with John.

Today we'd see if he could feed himself. I sat down beside him and opened the carton of orange juice. I inserted a straw and placed it in the left front corner of his tray. I showed it to him, told him what it was, and then placed the carton in his left hand and the straw in his mouth. He drank some, smiled, enjoying the taste of it, and put it back. He lifted it again, drank more and again returned it to the same location on the tray. Repeating this action several times, he finished the orange juice. Victory! He can feed himself. A giant leap of faith, I soon discovered.

I moved the empty juice carton out of his way and replaced it with the yogurt. Opening the container and stirring the yogurt with a plastic spoon, I told him what it was. I fed him one bite and put the spoon in his hand, leaving the yogurt on the front left corner of the tray.

"Now, you eat it," I told him.

John put the spoon back in the yogurt and picked up the container. He inserted the long, narrow end of the spoon into his mouth as if it were a straw, and tried to suck on it, just as he had done with the orange juice and the straw. Puzzled, I took it back, fed him another bite, handed him the spoon again and returned the yogurt to the tray.

Again, John replaced the spoon in the yogurt, picked up the container, and began sucking on the wrong end of the spoon. I repeated my actions. He repeated his. The third time I took it away, he got very annoyed, acting as if I were refusing to let him eat.

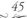

I was shocked by his bizarre behavior. How could he not know what a spoon was? How could he think it was a straw? He saw it. He found it easily on his tray. I simply couldn't understand what was happening. Stunned, I fed him the rest of his meal, afraid to risk upsetting him.

That was my first encounter with "perseveration", a characteristic of some stroke survivors, where the brain gets locked into a word or action and can't "change gears". I had only recently encountered the word and at first mistook it for "perseverance", but it was completely different. Books described it as a tendency to persist with the same response even though the stimulus has changed. John's brain was still telling him to sip from a straw even though he was holding a spoon in his hand. I had read about it with regard to communication difficulties, but hadn't understood the magnitude of the problem. I realized that I had no idea what was going on inside his brain and it scared me. Both John and I had a lot to learn.

A couple of times over the next few days, a physical therapist came to see John, to exercise his leg and arm. The sessions lasted only a few minutes and John, though amiable, was not responsive. I thought about his perseveration. Since John seemed to get locked into a response once he started doing something, I thought he might be able to move his leg if someone got him started. Perhaps it was naive, but I didn't know what else to do, and we had a lot of time. He was already showing some slight self-initiated movement in his foot and ankle.

While he was lying in bed, I would remove his sheet and slide his foot up and down along the surface of the bed, bending his knee in the process, as I had seen the therapists do. I would repeat it twenty or thirty times, up and down, up and down, and then tell him that I was going to let go and he was to keep doing it when I said, "ready, set, go." In the beginning, he simply stopped, but we kept trying. Finally, on the second day, he continued the movement alone. He was lying in bed, moving his leg up and down, on his own, perhaps five or six times. I was in heaven! Calling the nurses over, we cheered John's triumph.

Over the next few days, we repeated this exercise over and over. He was unable to initiate this leg movement, but once the routine was started, he usually kept it going. Encouraged by these results, I tried the same thing with his hand. I would open his fingers, then close them, over and over. I would lift his arm at the elbow, then lower it, over and over. There was a slight response, a slight uncurling of his fist, a slight lift of his arm, but nothing nearly so dramatic as his leg. But we kept at it, and John always received high praise for the smallest success. My sons had learned from me years before at their soccer games that every teammate's success earned a shout of congratulations, and every missed attempt an encouraging "good try". John's efforts deserved no less.

The step-down unit was kept uncomfortably warm. John wore a hospital gown, opened in the back and affording little privacy. The gown would usually ride up while he was in bed. Because of the heat, he was constantly kicking off his covers, and I, or someone else, was just as constantly covering him up. He seemed unaware of the impropriety of the situation, and by the end of the week, his nephew Thomas had affectionately dubbed him the Brooklyn flasher. One evening, while I was alone with him, and he had been constantly kicking off his sheet, his niece Courtney came to visit. Courtney was in her early twenties. I asked her to wait in the hallway for a minute.

"John, you have a visitor. It's your niece Courtney. She isn't used to seeing you naked and I don't want her to see you that way. She would be embarrassed. You *must* keep your covers on. This sheet has to stay here." I demonstrated where the cover had to stay, up around his chest.

"Do you want her to come in?"

John nodded.

"Then you'd better keep your covers on. Do you understand?" I tried to sound stern.

Again he nodded, though I wasn't at all sure he understood. Courtney entered the room and sat on the chair beside him. I perched at the end of the bed, ready to cover him quickly if necessary. We visited for a while. John was nodding and laughing as Courtney talked. Suddenly he looked at me, with a devilish glint in his eye, grabbed his sheet with his left hand, and with a jerking motion, flipped the cover down about a foot, and then back up again, and burst out laughing.

I was stunned! Not only had John understood, he had made a joke! He was teasing us. I was elated. His sense of humor was there, and though he was unable to communicate with words, his actions clearly conveyed the humor. This was my highlight of the two weeks at Maimonides. Humor had always gotten us through our most difficult times. The John I knew was somewhere inside this man. With humor we would bring him out. I left that night happier than I had been in a long time.

I was nervous about my visit to Kernan on Tuesday. The woman I met was sympathetic and understanding. Telling me about the rehabilitation schedule, she said that twice each day, patients met for thirty minutes with a speech therapist, a physical therapist, an occupational therapist, and once with a recreational therapist. Three and a half hours of therapy daily. Patients stayed from one to four weeks, rarely longer.

The facility was new, modern and immaculately clean. We toured the stroke unit. The patients were older than John, but most of them were walking and seemed very aware of their surroundings. In the adjacent Traumatic Brain Injury unit, a locked ward, patients were strapped into their wheelchairs. I didn't think to ask why we toured this wing, assuming it was just part of the tour, interesting but not relevant. I assumed that since John had a stroke, he would be admitted into the stroke unit.

Returning to her office, I felt torn between needing to tell this woman that John was much worse than the people I saw here, and being afraid that if I told her how bad he really was, they wouldn't admit him. I opted for honesty without full disclosure.

"All these people seem to be much better than John. I don't think John could figure out how to use a wheelchair. I'm not sure he could stay awake long enough for all that therapy. And four weeks isn't nearly long enough. I think it will be months before he's well enough to come home."

"John's head is still bandaged from the surgery. He doesn't seem to know what happened. I don't know if John knows who I am. He's never said anyone's name. I'm not sure he knows who he is."

My resolve to be strong was weakening. I hated that watery feeling behind my eyes, the thickness in my throat when I tried to speak. I was vulnerable and needed this woman's help. Would they take someone like John?

She said that sometimes they do admit a patient who is not ready for the rehabilitation program. When that happens, the patient may be temporarily moved into the University of Maryland hospital until he or she is recovered enough to participate in the therapy.

Kernan was a thirty-minute drive from our house. The commute between New York and Maryland was getting old quickly. I wanted John to be close to home. Kernan was modern and clean, didn't have a hospital smell and was covered under our insurance plan. John had to be out of Maimonides in three days. There were probably a hundred questions I should have asked, but I didn't know what they were. I only had one. Would they admit him?

She needed to talk to the doctors in the wards and they needed to talk with Dr. Anant. She would call me back, hopefully on Wednesday. I told her that Maimonides wanted to release him on Friday. Kathleen had located an ambulance service that would transport him to Baltimore. John's caseworker had said that our insurance would cover the move.

Wednesday Kernan called to say that John would be admitted to the Traumatic Brain Injury (TBI) Unit since John's condition was more similar to a traumatic brain injury than to a stroke. The ward was locked so patients couldn't wander off and get lost. Patients were strapped into their wheelchairs to reduce the chance of hurting themselves. I was relieved but surprised. Most of the people there were young men injured in car or bicycle accidents, some had gunshot wounds. It hadn't occurred to me that John had a traumatic brain injury. I was still adjusting to the word stroke. Hearing the term "traumatic brain injury" applied to John caused my stomach muscles to knot, it sounded so violent, and for some reason, more permanent. Couldn't they use gentler words?

There I was, getting hung up on labels again. The reality was bad enough, no matter what they called it. I knew what John was like. Attaching words to his condition didn't change him. At least Kernan thought they could help or they wouldn't have agreed to admit him. I hoped he could hack it. I didn't know where else to turn.

Wednesday morning, while I was driving up from Maryland, the doctors had scheduled John for Magnetic Resonance Imaging of his brain. Kathleen had gone with him as orderlies wheeled him to the basement MRI unit. When they tried to move him into the claustrophobic, drum-like tunnel, he panicked. Kathleen hovered over him, trying to calm him down and hold him still, unable to reason with him. Eventually, they gave up, unable to do the scans with John's constant motion.

I arrived at Maimonides early Wednesday afternoon and announced that John would be admitted to Kernan. Kathleen decided that she would ride with John in the ambulance from Maimonides to Kernan. I had to drive my car back. Mary and Steve would drive down to take Kathleen back home. Strictly speaking, it wasn't necessary, paramedics would be with him during the trip, but I knew they needed to feel okay about Kernan. They were reluctant to let John get so far away from them. They still didn't know very much about me, didn't know how well John would be taken care of, couldn't trust me yet with their brother's life. I could understand that. They were as worried about him as I was. I knew we would see them again soon, but it would be in Maryland, not Brooklyn. I felt guilty when Kathleen told me about John's reaction to the MRI, determined that next time I would be there for him. It would be so good to be home.

Friday afternoon, armed with nothing more than a pink discharge slip, and the doctor's phone number, we departed Maimonides. The trip took almost four hours. Our caravan arrived about five o'clock, exactly two weeks after John's stroke. It was time for a new beginning.

7

Our New Beginning

John was wheeled in on a stretcher to his new room in the Traumatic Brain Injury unit and transferred into a bed. This room was almost as large as the four-bed step-down unit at Maimonides but had only two beds and the other was unoccupied. We were pleased to learn from a nurse that there were no immediate plans for John to have a roommate. The window beside his bed opened to a courtyard and sunlight was streaming in. What a contrast from the view of a brick wall only a few feet from his last window! His room was clean and new, with no hospital smell. It seemed more like a spa. His private bathroom was spacious, with a large walk-in (probably wheel-in) shower. He had closet space, drawers, and his own TV, controlled by buttons on his bed rail. Another button rang at the nurses' station.

Kathleen, Mary and Steve looked delighted by his new surroundings. I was relieved by their reaction. It was important to me that they thought this place was okay. I wanted them to know that I had found a good place for John to recover. Getting John closer to home meant getting my life closer to normal, and if there was one thing I needed, it was to feel almost normal again. As much as I needed their approval, I needed to feel a measure of control returning to my life. I wanted the "home advantage".

Dr. Michael Makley, the medical director of the TBI unit, would be John's doctor during his stay at Kernan. He arrived within minutes of John's being settled in bed and introduced himself to us. Dr. Makley was a young man, about 5'11" with a slim build and a dark brown beard. He radiated a high energy level, moving swiftly, speaking quickly. He asked to see John's paperwork. I showed him the pink piece of paper from Maimonides with the word "discharge" written boldly across the form and silently resolved in the future to do a better job of getting hospital paperwork. This was clearly the abbreviated version of his medical records.

John was awake and smiling, but looked tired. The bandage on his head had been removed that morning at Maimonides. Much of the already thinning gray hair on the top and left side of his head had been shaved for the surgery, leaving some very uneven hair on the sides and top. The rest was just beginning to grow back, short and stubby. A large red scar crossed with bold black stitches stretched from the top of his head, beside his crown, curving down behind his left ear—about five or six inches long. A significant dent interrupted the scar where the surgeon had entered his skull. Because of the surgery, his hair hadn't been washed in two weeks. I had adjusted to the way John looked, but trying to see him as a stranger would, I realized he looked pretty awful.

Dr. Makley began to examine John. "Hello, John. I'm Dr. Makley. How are you feeling today?" he asked in a commanding voice.

His question had gotten John's attention. Since his stroke, John's voice had become much softer, in marked contrast to his stronger voice from before. John winced at the loud sounds, eyed him cautiously and nodded, but made no other response.

Dr. Makley turned to me. "Does he know who he is?"

"I think so, but I'm not sure."

Turning again to John, he explained to him that he was at Kernan, that he was going to examine him, that John was going to be staying there while he got better. As the examination proceeded, John was cooperative but clearly didn't understand what Dr. Makley said to him. Each instruction, "sit up", "breathe deeply", "look at me", "follow my finger", each question, "Can you tell me your name?", "Do you know what happened to you?" was acknowledged with a nod and a smile, but no other action or response.

Dr. Makley looked at me. "So what can you tell me?"

I was anxious to tell him what I knew. As Kathleen, Mary and Steve listened, I spoke quickly, just as he had. I described John's pre-stroke condition, the circumstances surrounding his stroke, his condition immediately before surgery, and what I knew of the surgery. I told him about a mysterious fever that John had his last few days at Maimonides, which seemed to have gone. I listed the tests that had been done, and which ones they had been unable to do. I told him that John was taking Dilantin, a medication to prevent seizures and that he was eating solid foods. I described his current capabilities with regard to his physical and mental condition, as I observed them.

"What is your home situation like? Are you working? What is your house like?"

I told him about John's three grown children and my two sons. His daughter Janet lived nearby with her husband and two children. My son David would probably be home from college for the summer, but otherwise, we lived alone. I told him about my company, that I traveled frequently, but had canceled most of the scheduled trips for the next several weeks to be here.

As for our house, it was not handicap-friendly. I admitted that it would present a hostile environment to a wheelchair-bound person, assuming that John could use a wheelchair. I described the architectural problems we would have with stairs, bathrooms, upstairs bedrooms, difficult entryways, narrow doors and the outside deck on three levels. Other things, rugs, furniture, were easier to move or remove.

Dr. Makley explained what John's schedule would be like. Since it was Friday evening, and the staff was light on Saturday, John might not be seen by all the therapists before Monday. Sunday was a day of rest and no therapy sessions were scheduled that day, so John might get two more days of rest before therapy began. I had mixed feelings. On the one hand, I wanted John to get started as soon as possible. On the other, having more time to adjust and recuperate might increase his likelihood of success.

Dr. Makley would see John daily, would be consulting with other doctors, particularly stroke specialists, who would also meet with John, and would be following his progress closely. The stroke unit was adjacent to the TBI. While it was somewhat unusual for a stroke survivor to be in this ward, it was also unusual for a person with a massive intracerebral hemorrhage to be a survivor. The doctors had discussed John's case and felt that, because of his significant disorientation and the severe trauma to his brain, this was where he should be. A caseworker at Kernan would be assigned to manage his case. I would meet her on Monday.

Starting Monday, John would receive at least 3½ hours of therapy every day. After he was evaluated by his therapists, they would establish weekly and long-term goals for John. They would set up a schedule for each day, one week at a time. Dr. Makley conducted weekly meetings with his staff to evaluate each patient's progress and they would inform me of John's results. I could visit John in the evenings, after therapy, and on weekends.

I interrupted. "Dr. Makley, I plan to attend as many of John's therapy sessions as I can. Everyday."

His reaction was guarded. "We discourage family members from visiting during the day. It can be disruptive to the patient. The patient needs to focus on getting better while he's here. Visitors can be distracting, both for the patient and the therapist."

"Doctor, I'm not a visitor, I'm his wife. I want John to get better, probably more than anyone else in the world. I promise I will not be disruptive or distracting. I don't know much about rehabilitation, but I need to learn. In a few weeks, he'll be coming home. I have as much to learn as John does. I promise not to get in the way. If I do, you can ask me to leave. But please, let me try."

"We'll see."

I took that to be a yes, unless John's therapists objected, and changed the subject.

I voiced my concerns about how much therapy John could handle, but stressed that I wanted him to get as much help as they could give him, and I would do everything I could to help. I was concerned that the four-week limit mentioned during the initial interview was not long enough. It was hard to believe that he could return home so soon. If he didn't know who he was, or who I was, did he have any concept of "home"? And could I take care of him alone?

Dr. Makley said that the length of the stay was usually limited by what the insurance company would pay, and even to stay four weeks would require visible progress by the patient and weekly authorizations from the insurance company. He suggested that we wait and see how John improved before determining how long he would stay. Realizing it was pointless to argue about when he would be discharged before the admissions procedures were even complete, I backed off.

Privately, I knew it wasn't only John I was worried about. John needed to stay until I was capable of taking care of him. Other than a stint as a Candy Striper in high school, I had no experience with sick people, no nursing skills beyond the motherly patching of skinned knees, and my medical education was now in its second week. I was afraid to move him from the bed to a chair for fear of hurting him and jumped to call a nurse every time a machine beeped in his room. I couldn't believe four weeks was long enough for either of us to learn what we needed to, to survive.

We spoke for a few more minutes before Dr. Makley left. Kathleen, Mary and Steve had a long drive back and needed to leave. I went out to meet the nurses while they said their good-byes.

Each nurse was assigned specific patients. Cheryl, the woman who would be John's primary nurse, introduced herself. I told her a little bit about him. I hated leaving him in the care of people who didn't know him, of people I didn't know. My experience with nurses was limited to my annual checkups, when they weighed you (heartlessly recording the exact weight, never giving you any credit for heavy clothing), took your blood pressure and were present during examinations.

The nurses here would be doing a lot more than that for John. It had to be a hard job. I didn't think I could take care of a stranger the way I wanted them to take care of John. I liked Cheryl right away, but it still scared me to just drop him off and leave, trusting that he would be watched and checked and not ignored. At Maimonides, he was surrounded by family at least sixteen hours a day, and at his family's direction, when he was moved out of the intensive care unit, I paid for a private nurse to sit beside his bed and watch him all night, apparently a common practice in New York. Here he was helpless.

Mary emerged teary-eyed from John's room. Though Mary, Steve and Kathleen all said how pleased they were with what they had seen, they had the same misgivings about leaving him there that I did. The big difference, I believed, was that their real, unspoken concern was leaving him with me. I understood that. I probably would have felt the same way had the tables been turned and I was leaving a brother in the hands of a wife I didn't know well. But I also knew that I would do everything I could for him. Trust takes time and we all needed a lot of it. With hugs, kisses, and promises to call, they left.

I returned to his room, sat down beside him and took his hand. He was all mine now. I felt so many conflicting emotions—relief that he was finally here in Maryland, a space we would share together in which he could begin to recover, relief that his family was gone and I was finally alone with him. But that aloneness brought fear—his family had been so good to us and would have been there to help if he'd stayed in New York. I believed I had made the right decision, hoped that these new surrounding would provide the help he needed. The only emotions that were blessedly absent, at least for the moment, were guilt and sadness.

Together we were facing the most incredible challenge of our lives. He needed all the support I could give him to help him get well again. Did he know who I was? He'd been treating everyone the same, with smiles and amiable cooperation, but no active participation. Did he even know what a wife was? What's going on inside his head? Can what's broken be fixed? What all is broken?

Is John scared? Does he understand enough to be scared? Could he tell me if he was? Is his brain somehow protecting him from being scared? I hoped that was true because I thought that if he understood what was going on, he should be terrified. I was scared for him. I wished over and over that I could see inside his brain and know what was going on in there.

He was so vulnerable, and so trusting. I wanted to protect him. I looked at John and he smiled. I smiled back and squeezed his hand. He squeezed mine. We were in this together. The John that was emerging was sweet, gentle, smiling, cheerful, and I felt good just being around him. I liked this gentle side of John and I liked being with this man. What we had right now felt pretty good and I was grateful for this moment. We sat there for a while as the sun began to set. I spoke quietly to him, telling him again where he was, how close to home he was and that I would leave soon, but would be back early the next day.

John was getting tired. I was tired too, but was already looking forward to tomorrow. It was time to leave. His nurse Cheryl showed me how to strap John into his bed, lock the strap, and hang the key across the room on the cork board where he couldn't reach it. She said this was a precaution taken with all patients. He might not realize he couldn't walk; he might fall out of bed and not be able to call for help. He could hurt himself. I hated doing it. Locking him in bed seemed so drastic, but I couldn't refuse and was surprised as I had been so often by his behavior in the past two weeks when John didn't seem to mind. I kissed him good-bye, promised to return in the morning and left.

Driving home, I thought again about how helpless he was. I didn't like leaving him in the hands of strangers who didn't know him, who didn't know who he had been before this tragedy occurred. At Maimonides, he slept most of the time. Now he was waking up. Here, they would see a man who didn't understand what they said to him, who couldn't follow the simplest verbal command, who seemed very pleasant, but confused. John couldn't walk, or talk, or feed himself. He was locked in his bed, couldn't summon help if he needed it, and couldn't complain. He was alone in his room. If they didn't care, it would be easy to ignore him. I wasn't ready to trust them.

Perhaps they would care more if they knew more about him. I decided to compose a background on John and present it to his caseworker, the doctor, his therapists, and his nurses so they would know who he was and who he could be again. I wanted them to care as much as I cared.

Arriving home, too preoccupied to eat, I went immediately to the computer and starting writing. By midnight I was satisfied that the two page background had summarized the essentials. I had a rule at my company: Know your audience and never write more than they will read, lest the entire document be filed away for "when there's more time", a future hour that usually doesn't arrive. I decided that two pages was the limit and it needed to tell them as much as possible about John Quann before his stroke—who he was, what he liked, how he lived. They needed to know he was a reader, a writer, a traveler, a biker, and jogger, a mathematician and engineer—a man full of life and humor. I hoped that when they read it, John would become more real to them and they would use the information to get inside his brain and help him get well again. Tired, as always lately, I went to bed and slept soundly.

I woke up refreshed and excited about having two whole days alone with John, satisfied that I had done something positive the night before to help him. I showered, dressed, and rushed to Kernan with five copies of John's background in a manila folder.

Pushing a button near the entrance unlocked the door to his ward. Once inside, the door could only be opened by the button hidden behind the nurses' station. It was weird to think of my husband in a locked hospital ward, but almost everything in this alien world seemed weird lately. John's door was open, but his room was empty. I panicked. Where was he? Had something happened during the night? Why hadn't they called me? I rushed to the nurses' station to discover that he was being evaluated by the physical therapist. Already? Where?

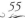

The nurse directed me to the PT room where John was lying on a mat on the floor, a young woman sitting beside him. John looked okay and smiled as if he recognized me. I greeted John and introduced myself to Susan, his physical therapist. She was tall and slim, smiling and friendly. She had been evaluating him.

"He doesn't seem to be able to move his leg," she stated.

"Yes, he can," I jumped in.

I explained what we had been doing at Maimonides and asked if I could show her. She agreed immediately. With John lying on his back, I started his leg moving up and down, over and over, as we had practiced and finally said, "Ready, set, go!" He continued the movement.

"John, that's wonderful, you're doing great," I said proudly. He looked pleased.

Susan was amazed and delighted. She hadn't been able to get him to move it alone. I told her that I wanted to attend as many of John's sessions as I could and if I got in the way, to please tell me and I'd back off. She had no problem with that. I handed her a copy of John's biography and asked her to read it when she could. She seemed surprised but pleased to get it and promised she would read it.

John's evaluation was just ending. She moved him into his wheelchair, directing him both orally and with gestures how to position himself as she did it. Susan impressed me as being very confident and capable, not at all afraid as I was to lift or move him. She praised him for his cooperation and told him that he was doing a great job.

He smiled and said, "Thank you. I appreciate it." I was startled. The words may have been part of his automatic speech, but they were sincere, and the most coherent and appropriate thing he had said in two weeks. Susan smiled and thanked him also. What a great start.

I was uncomfortable as she strapped John into the wheelchair, using a long, wide fabric belt that reminded me of the belts my boys had worn in their karate lessons years ago.

"Why do you have to do that?" I asked.

"For his own protection. He might forget that he can't walk and try to get up. Patients here can be very disoriented. Whenever he's alone, he needs to be strapped in. The first goal for all patients is safety, the second is rehabilitation."

A locked ward, restraints that locked him in bed at night and strapped him in a wheelchair by day—I'd go crazy if they did that to me, but at the moment John didn't seem to mind. Maybe she was right but it conjured up images of mental institutions and dangerous people. Was John dangerous to himself? Were other people dangerous? Could someone hurt John?

Susan showed me the safety features of the wheelchair, how to lock and unlock the wheels, how to strap him in so he could not get out. She located and attached an armrest to the right side of his wheelchair and demonstrated how to rest his right arm on it to avoid injuring his shoulder. She told me that I would be trained later to help him move in and out of his wheelchair— "wheelchair transfers", Susan called them. I walked beside them as she wheeled him back to his room. She told him she would see him on Monday and left.

No other therapists were scheduled to see him that day. John looked tired, but the nurse said that lunch would be arriving in an hour and suggested that he wait until after lunch to take a nap, so we began to explore his new surroundings. After we checked out his room, his TV, bathroom, closet and drawers, we went to the nurses' station. I gave them a copy of John's background and asked them to read it and put it in his file. As I wheeled him around the unit, we explored, discovering together where things were. I talked to him about what we were seeing. I tried to show him how to move the wheelchair himself, but he was too tired, too weak, or simply didn't understand. In any event, he wasn't able to make it move.

When lunch arrived, I fed him, letting him drink by himself using a straw. That he could do. He was eating well and clearly enjoyed mealtime. Before his stroke, John had been very particular about what he ate. Now he devoured every bite with relish. Fortunately, the meals at Kernan were pretty good, but his enthusiasm surprised me—most of it he wouldn't have touched three weeks ago. Even Jell-O got his resounding approval. Watching the pleasure he got from eating was fun in itself.

I wondered if he would maintain the same level of enthusiasm for eating when he got home. Clearly my mashed potatoes were far superior to theirs. Mine had garlic and sour cream. Could he tell the difference or was everything wonderful? Would he now condescend to eat an occasional dinner of macaroni and cheese, that artery-clogging, heart attack-inducing meal only a wife bent on homicide would consider serving him? The thought amused me. Boy, would that make life easier!

Nap time. A nurse came to transfer him into his bed. She removed his shoes, tucked him in under the sheet and strapped him in—my mind revolted against the strapping in part, but it was the rule. Within minutes, he was asleep.

It would be a couple of hours before he would wake up. He needed some clothes that were easy to put on and take off. I drove to the nearby Wal-Mart and purchased a few pairs of soft cotton knit shorts and pants with elastic waists, clothes he wouldn't have been caught dead in before.

John had always been meticulous about his dental hygiene. Each night he used to brush his teeth with a regular toothbrush, floss for about ten minutes, then brush again with an electric toothbrush. Until a few days ago, he'd had a tube down his throat. I didn't know if anyone had brushed his teeth since his stroke. I knew he hadn't flossed. He only had one good arm but I didn't think I could floss for him, and the idea held little appeal for me. I found dental floss on picks that he could use with one hand. Worth a try. Armed with a toothbrush, toothpaste, dental floss and new clothes, I returned to Kernan.

John was awake and sitting up in bed with the TV on. Someone had checked on him, a good sign. Cheryl was on duty and when she came into the room, she had already read John's brief biography. God bless her.

We chatted for a couple of minutes. I showed her the things I had just bought for John.

"Do you think he'd like to take a shower?" she asked.

"He'd love it! Can you give him a shower? Can I help? What about his head?"

"Sure you can help. We'll just be careful with his head."

She closed the door and cheerfully asked John if he would like to take a shower. He smiled and nodded. John seemed good at reading body language and my excitement probably carried over. I doubt he understood what was about to transpire, but if we looked happy about it, it must be okay. We undressed him and she transferred him into the wheelchair. When the water was warm enough, she wheeled him into the bathroom.

I removed my shoes and socks, rolled up my jeans and shirt sleeves, ready to join in the adventure. Cheryl transferred him to a shower chair. Using a hand-held shower spray, she began spraying warm water all over him. John radiated delight, grinning and almost moaning in pleasure. We cleaned him with soapy washcloths. Cheryl cleaned his hair that I had been afraid to touch. I wondered ironically if John thought he'd died and gone to heaven. Knowing how good it felt to take a shower when you're sick, a shower after two weeks confined to a hospital bed must feel soothingly luxurious. John would have let the shower continue forever, but eventually it had to end. John looked at Cheryl as if she wore a halo, smiled again and said, "Thank you. I appreciate it."

That's twice. A fluent, coherent and appropriately grateful response. It turned out to be about the only one he had and he repeated it frequently and sincerely to everyone—the luck of the Irish I decided, as he soon won the entire staff over with it.

After Cheryl dressed John, she said it would be okay to take him outside after his hair dried. She showed me where to sign him out and said that he could leave the ward with me anytime, as long as he didn't have any scheduled activities. We could go to the courtyard outside his window or to the front of the building, where we could catch the sun in the late afternoon. Cheryl was wonderful.

I wheeled John outside to soak in the late afternoon sun and we held hands while I talked to him. He seemed so happy, so relaxed, so content. Food, a shower, the warm afternoon sun, John's pleasures were simple and uncomplicated.

He held my hand as if he cherished it. I felt good being with him, not angry, not sad, just grateful that he seemed so happy to be alive, glad that he seemed so happy to be with me. We were lucky. These special moments together in the late afternoon were to become an important part of every day at Kernan.

We went back inside for dinner. Again, he relished every bite. By seven o'clock, he was falling asleep. Cheryl came in, prepared him for bed and locked him in. When he fell asleep, I left.

Sunday morning I was feeling brave and nervous. I had decided to bring in his electric razor. At Maimonides, the nurses had shaved him. Would he know what a razor was? Actually I had a bigger concern. Dr. Anant told us that John's vision had been damaged. The medical term was a "complete homonymous hemianopsia". In laymen's terms, I understood it to mean that John could see out of the left half of both eyes and nothing out of the right half of either eye. Effectively, his field of view began directly in front of him and extended fully to the left. He saw nothing to the right of him from either eye. His visual field was cut in half. Something on his right would only come into his field of view as it passed directly in front of him, or when he turned his head to the right.

The medical literature described "neglect" as a neurological disorder, where the patient ignores, or neglects one side of his body. This could accompany his visual deficit. In its more severe forms, a person could ignore his paralysis, deny it, or not even acknowledge that the paralyzed limbs are his. They simply ignore half of their bodies. The literature described women who applied lipstick to only one side of their lips, men who shaved only one side of their faces. John couldn't see anything to his right. He didn't see people, food on his tray, objects in his way. Prognosis for physical recovery was diminished for patients with severe neglect. I had mixed feelings about this experiment, but I might as well know. This was not the kind of problem that would go away if one ignored it. Besides, when he couldn't feed himself, I'd fed him. If he couldn't shave, I could learn to do that too. Please God, just let this one thing work, I found myself asking again.

John perked up when I walked into the room. Maybe he does know who I am. Both that thought and just seeing John again cheered me. I greeted him with a hug and a kiss. How could you not feel good when someone looked so pleased to see you? He was already dressed and in his wheelchair. I showed him the toothbrush, dental floss and razor. I held the razor to his face, reminded him how to use it and wheeled him into the bathroom, positioning him in front of the sink and mirror.

John hadn't seen himself in a mirror since his stroke. Initially he looked too horrible and I was afraid it would upset him. Later, the opportunity hadn't presented itself and I'd just forgotten. How he looked hadn't seemed nearly as important as what he understood or how he felt.

He stared at himself. Touching his right cheek where it drooped, he looked at his face. He looked at his semi-shaved head and at the dark ugly red scar. His hand moved near the scar, but he didn't touch it. He seemed startled, surprised, curious, afraid. He looked pained, not as though it hurt, but as though it had happened to someone else and he felt sorry for that person. It was as though he had empathy for the person in the mirror, as if it were another person, not John. He must have stared for a full two minutes as I waited silently. Was he beginning to understand that he was the man in the mirror?

Time for the scary part now. I handed him the electric razor and turned it on. What would he do with it? Using his left hand, he began shaving the left side of his face. He knew what it was! Thank God. I backed away and stood by the door, out of his field of view, letting him shave by himself, trying to act calm and natural. Watching from several feet away, I prayed he would shave his whole face. Silently my mind willed him to move the razor to the right side of his face. Yes! Yes! Awkwardly he shaved his right cheek, his neck, his chin. He did see his whole face! At least physically, he saw the man in the mirror. Another victory—thank you, God. Watching John shave was so exciting. It sure beat watching him sleep!

His only frustration seemed to stem from the awkwardness of shaving with his left hand, but I was too relieved to be sympathetic and said he'd have to get used to it, and it would get easier with practice. Next came the toothbrush. I applied toothpaste and handed it to him. Using his left hand, he brushed his teeth. I was pushing my luck with the dental floss, but handed it to him anyway. I took one and explained what it was, then used it to floss my own teeth. He must have seen it before and recognized it, or understood what to do, because he used it correctly. It struck me as ironic that flossing was more instinctive than eating, dental floss more recognizable than a spoon, removing food from his mouth more automatic than putting it in. I doubted that would have been the case for me.

Sunday was a quiet day. He ate. We talked—mostly I talked, since there was almost nothing John could say. John seemed unaware that most of his speech was gibberish. We went outside. He wanted to know more about what had happened to him. He indicated this by pointing to his head, and with a puzzled expression said, "What...?" Each time I told him the story about his stroke, it was as if he had not heard it before. I believed that he understood some, but not most of what I said to him, when I said it. He knew something had happened. He grimaced when I described the headache, the hospital, the surgery. He listened so hard, trying to concentrate, to understand. He touched me a lot, rubbing my hand and my arm, as though he needed the physical contact. I reciprocated. We held hands and smiled. It was easy to tell him that everything would be okay, that he was getting better. I believed it.

John was tired. He would need all his energy the next day to participate in the full schedule of therapy. Returning to his room, I watched the nurse prepare him for bed, offered him a choice of CDs that I had brought from home, and sat beside his bed as he listened to the religious chants that he selected. He fell asleep holding my hand, looking so gentle, so vulnerable. But I'd seen enough of John sleeping to last a long time. Now that he had settled in, it was time to start working.

8

"Slowly But Surely"—Recovering the Body

Monday morning after stopping by my office, I arrived at Kernan about ten o'clock to find John in the physical therapy area riding a stationary bicycle. I was stunned and terrified. John can't do that! He's paralyzed! He'll hurt himself! What can they be thinking?

Then I spotted Susan watching from a few feet away while John sat on the bicycle. She had tied his right hand to the bicycle handle and his right foot to the pedal. He was pedaling, using his left foot for momentum. He wouldn't stop. Perseveration perhaps, but John was beaming. He looked so proud of himself. Susan was beaming. She had read in John's biography that he was an experienced and enthusiastic biker and thought that getting him on a bicycle might stimulate his legs. She had set the timer for five minutes. John didn't want to stop. Ten, fifteen, twenty minutes passed. Finally she stopped him, afraid he would be too exhausted to do anything else for the rest of the day. John stopped reluctantly. He probably would have continued until he collapsed.

Over the next few days, he began to understand how to make the wheelchair move. Using only his left hand, moving in a straight direction was difficult, but he persisted. His right hand would often slide off the armrest and someone would replace it, not wanting to add a dislocated shoulder to the rest of his problems. Eventually, he began to lift his paralyzed right hand with his left to place it back on the armrest when he was reminded. But it was as if he were helping someone else, as if this appendage were somehow attached and detached at the same time.

Throughout his weeks at Kernan, John amazed me every day, either because of what he could do, or because of what he could not. So many things were going on in parallel during those four weeks. In my mind, his recovery had two components—the physical and the cognitive. It is easier to focus on his physical recovery first because he made so much progress there. It could be measured daily, in one case hourly. Nothing was easy, but almost everything was successful and every accomplishment felt like a giant step forward.

From the beginning, John showed a determination to get well. Not that any of us understood fully what that meant, but he seemed to understand his physical limitations and could focus on them. Each day in physical therapy, Susan would push him harder than I thought he could go. And John would try.

At first, she had him climbing a ladder. As she held him up, she placed one foot on the first rung and his left hand on a rung above his head. She would urge him to pull himself up to the next rung. I sat on the edge of my chair watching, terrified that he would fall, that she would not be able to catch him if he fell. And he would struggle. She would sit him down to rest. After a few seconds, he would say, "One more time," and attempt to get up, to try again.

As the days passed, Susan had John balancing himself on huge balls, rolling on a mat, moving from a lying to a sitting position, from sitting to standing. He was exercising on a stationary bike and awkwardly climbing a ladder. She was right beside him, helping him, holding him, ready to catch him before he could fall. I was always afraid, afraid he would fall, afraid she was pushing him beyond his limits, and secretly I guess, afraid he would fail at each new task, afraid he would become discouraged. But John pushed himself even harder than Susan did, and he left each session exhausted, pleased with himself and grateful to her.

Learning to walk again was laborious and exhausting. With Susan on one side of John and an assistant on the other, they would lift him upright, move one foot and then the other. God, it looked so hard. After one or two steps, Susan would sit John down and tell him to rest. Beads of sweat covered his face from the sheer exertion. After a couple of seconds, he would look at her and say, "One more time."

They would lift him up again and help him take a couple more steps. He would be grimacing when they sat him down to rest.

Each time, he looked at her with determination. "One more time," he repeated again.

And they did it one more time. Each day, each time, he did a little more himself. Each time when she sat him down to rest, obviously in pain, obviously exhausted, he would look at her with sheer determination and say, "One more time."

I felt torn between being so proud of him and yet wanting to cry for the pain he was feeling. How could he do this to himself? It was so hard. If he approached each difficult task with that same single-minded determination, I knew he would recover as much as he possibly could.

Finally, when each session was over, John would smile at Susan and say, "Thank you. I appreciate it." He would look at me with a grin and say with pleasure in his voice, "Slowly but surely." It was as if he knew with certainty that he would walk again.

While John met twice each day with Susan, his physical therapist, he also met twice daily with Janet, his occupational therapist (OT). Janet's job involved exercising the top half of his body, principally his arm and hand, and working on thinking skills that did not involve speech. As OT, Janet was also responsible for "Activities for Daily Living", ADLs. These included skills like dressing, bathing and eating. After reading John's background, she discovered that her father, who had worked at Goddard, knew John. She was a sweet, soft-spoken, very pretty young woman and seemed to enjoy working with John. He was always cheerful, motivated and trying hard to understand the task at hand. She treated him with respect and enthusiasm and they both seemed to light up during the time they spent together.

It was difficult for John to dress himself because of his paralyzed right side, but it was not perplexing. By that I mean, he needed help getting clothes on and off, but he understood that labels went in the back of shirts and pants and that socks went on under shoes, not the other way around. Strange to feel grateful for that, but I had read that it was not uncommon to confuse such things. He didn't seem to care much about what he wore, content with whatever was offered to him. Except he liked to have his cardigan sweater with him. Was he cold, or anticipating getting cold, or was it the only item of clothing he recognized as his own, his old wardrobe now replaced with soft, easy to wear sweats? Regardless, his cardigan went everywhere with him.

Regaining control over his bathroom functions was an important part of his physical recovery. Being tied in a wheelchair, it was obviously not something he could do alone. Initially, he would become agitated after an accident, but it was not clear whether he was unable to express his need, or simply didn't realize it. Several strategies were tried to enable John to "tell" someone. He couldn't point to a bathroom. Often there was no bathroom in sight. He couldn't say the word bathroom. He couldn't reliably answer a yes/no question, so asking him didn't have much success.

One of his speech therapists developed a communication board (a plastic covered piece of paper divided into twelve squares, each square containing a picture of something he might need—a toilet, a bed, a sweater, a drink, food, pencil and paper, etc.) and taped it to the armrest on his wheelchair. But he could not use it to point to the picture of the toilet because, as we came to discover in his speech sessions, he was unable to associate an object with a picture of the object.

So, he was taken to the bathroom a few times a day, when someone else decided it might be time. This worked to the extent that his body cooperated with a nurse's schedule. Obviously, it was not a perfect system. If he became agitated, I sometimes correctly guessed at the problem, other times I did not. Then one day, out of the blue, he looked at me and said, "I have to pee."

What a beautiful sentence! Fortunately it turned out to be a repeatable one. Two days later, after a perfect record of success, Cheryl suggested he was ready for regular underwear. That night, as he was getting ready for bed, I held up a pair of briefs.

"How would you like to wear these?" I asked with a grin.

In a voice filled with wonder and hope, he responded, "Do you think I can?"

God, how I loved his few whole sentences! They allowed me to forget, even for a few seconds, where we were and why we were here.

"Yes, I think you can. But if you have an accident, it's not the end of the world. Would you like to try?"

John's nod was a definite yes, and it was the last time we had to worry about it. Another major victory, another giant step forward.

"It's not the end of the world" was a phrase I used often and it helped keep things in perspective. My mother had said it hundreds of times as her seven children were growing up. Whether applied to spilled milk or major life catastrophes, it was her pragmatic way of dealing with life's upsets. It was a phrase that would be passed down to future generations in my family. I once overheard my four-year-old niece calmly decree it when her brother had broken a flower vase. It wasn't something you could argue with. It placed no blame. It simply accepted what was. Comparing life's mishaps with the end of the world made them seem pretty inconsequential. John was alive and recovering. The rest we could deal with.

Movement in John's right hand was coming back, but more slowly than his leg and foot. Janet would exercise his hand during his OT sessions with her. She showed me how to do it. Together, John and I would work on it outside of his sessions, squeezing, pinching, touching fingers. But he could not lift his arm. John ate with his left hand, but as his right hand began to get some movement back, I sometimes put a spoon in his right hand to see if he could eat with it.

He was unsuccessful until April 7, almost four weeks after his stroke. His son Christopher had flown in from Salt Lake City to visit him that day. At breakfast, resting his arm on the table, he held the spoon in his right hand, dipped the spoon into his breakfast cereal and lowered his head to the spoon. His first right-handed bite! By lunch, his arm was a couple of inches off the table as he ate. By dinner, he was lifting it almost six inches and lowering his head only slightly. Not only was this a major victory, to me it was a miracle. He had made incredible progress in a single day. It was as if his arm had gently awakened. Apparently, in the four weeks that had elapsed since his surgery, enough of the swelling in his brain had gone down and enough of the blood

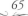
had receded in the area of his brain that controlled this movement to regain use. It encouraged our hope for further recovery, and hope kept us going.

In Janet's OT sessions, John was sorting variously shaped objects and inserting them into the right holes, assembling simple puzzles, and working with equipment to strengthen his hand muscles. He rarely understood a task when it was first explained to him, but he could usually succeed after being shown once or twice how to do it. Each task was designed to strengthen his right hand and arm. Janet would often ask me to sit beside him and hold his left hand to prevent him from using it during these exercises. Though the tasks were often difficult for him, he always tried hard and seemed more curious than frustrated by the behavior of his limb. He left each session with a smile, saying, "Thank you, I appreciate it."

The first week John was at Kernan, I scheduled an appointment with an architect who specialized in handicapped accommodations. The stairs were particularly worrisome since the bedrooms and full baths were on the second floor. Our home might require major renovations. After two weeks at Kernan, John was taking a few hesitant steps alone, still always with Susan beside him, to grab him if he started to fall. Twice, I rescheduled the appointment with the architect, seeing progress so quickly, unsure what would need to be done. By his fourth week there, as Susan was preparing him to return home, they practiced walking up and down the stairs. Now, as long as I or someone else was with him, he did not need to be strapped into the wheelchair. He could stand up and take a few steps by himself, though most of his day was still spent in the wheelchair.

John's friend Art dropped by to visit him at least once a week. Art didn't treat John like he was sick. Art treated him like he was John. One evening, during John's fourth week, when I had a business function to attend, my sister Annie spent the evening with John. Art came to visit. Sitting, but no longer strapped into his wheelchair, since Annie was with him, John carefully got up and walked several steps across the room to get something. Progress had been so rapid and Art hadn't seen John for a several days. Annie didn't realize that Art didn't know that John could walk. Art, eyes bulging and mouth dropping open, thought he was witnessing a miracle. A *real* miracle. The next day, for my benefit, John imitated Art's reaction and laughed over it for days.

Dr. Makley scheduled John to have an MRI two days before he left Kernan. A specially equipped van transported us to the University of Maryland Medical Center in downtown Baltimore. It was John's first trip off the grounds at Kernan. The van deposited us at the front entrance. With a nurse and myself beside him, John walked the lengths of the hospital halls pushing his wheelchair. His walk was slow but steady and otherwise normal. He didn't look like the same patient who only a few weeks before had been strapped and locked in that chair. This time the MRI went smoothly. That evening I canceled the appointment with the architect. Our house was no longer the physical obstacle it had been.

The day before he left Kernan, Susan took him into the swimming pool. She had promised him that they would do it and John had been anticipating it with enthusiasm and fear. Regretfully, I missed the event but realized as soon as I arrived that morning that something special had happened. John was beaming.

"I did it! I did it!" he almost pounced on me when I arrived, barely able to contain himself in the wheelchair to which he was strapped.

"Did what? What did you do?" I laughed. He was so excited. He couldn't wait to tell me.

He motioned by stretching his arm over his head, hand arching down, his face down, a swimming motion, interjecting gibberish as he rushed to demonstrate.

"You went swimming?"

"Yes, yes," he nodded excitedly.

"How was it? Could you swim?"

"I was great!"

He used gestures to describe what had happened. From his charades, my questions, and his responses, I gathered that he had swum the length of the pool, that he was surprised to discover that his right arm had seemed very weak when he lifted it out of the water with each overhand stroke, and that he was very proud of himself. That afternoon Susan confirmed that the adventure had been a success, that his right arm had been heavy in the water, but John could swim. John's abundant gratitude towards Susan was evident, as he thanked her over and over.

On his last morning, his last session with Susan, she took him outside to the front of the building. There was a long six-foot-wide concrete handicap ramp that connected the parking lot with the entrance to the building. She knew that John had been a jogger, that he liked to run. She walked down with him to the bottom of the ramp and told him they were going to run up the ramp. He looked surprised. She moved to stand beside him, bent down, positioning herself as at the start of a race. He understood. She was going to race beside him. John grinned and got in position.

"Ready, set, GO!" she called. And off they went. John thought he was flying and though his perception of speed didn't quite match reality, he was thrilled. He was triumphant!

John remembered those two events, swimming and running up the handicap ramp vividly. For months afterwards, to the extent that he could tell his story, he retold them, over and over again. To John, they must have represented freedom and independence and success. They were his major milestones, perhaps more significant to him than the stroke itself, of which he rarely spoke.

During John's four weeks at Kernan, his physical recovery was astonishing. Much credit goes to Susan and Janet, his therapists, much to John's sheer determination to get well, much to the amazing recovery powers of the mind and body, much to his support system of family and friends, and I give God his fair share. I believe that hard work and miracles can go together. Perhaps the fact that he was willing to work so hard was part of the miracle.

$\approx$ 9 $\approx$

Aphasia—The Cognitive Challenge

I wish I could have understood what was going on inside John's head in those four weeks at Kernan. I could observe it, but clearly, I could not understand it. John had aphasia. I had never heard the word before, and wasn't even sure I was pronouncing it right when I first read about it (uh-FAY-zhia). Speech-Language Pathology books define it as a language disorder, caused by brain injury in which one or more aspects of language comprehension and language production may be affected. The American Heart Association notes that people with aphasia may have trouble speaking, understanding, reading or writing. The National Institute of Health estimates that 85,000 new cases of aphasia occur every year and that more than one million Americans have some form of it. The severity and the symptoms of aphasia are different for every person. Books and medical articles document technical aspects of it and proposed treatments for specific problems. There is no medical cure. Although rehabilitation offers some hope, full recovery of language and cognition after a severe stroke is unusual.

In John's case, the aphasia was severe and encompassed a wide range of symptoms. To the extent that I could distance myself from it and observe it clinically, I would say that John's aphasia was both incredibly bizarre and fascinating. As a wife however, I was frightened, frustrated and confused. I feared for John's isolation and felt overwhelmingly protective. I shared the mother lion's response—no one was going to hurt my John. I knew he was safe at Kernan, but that would not always be true.

I have described John's physical recovery during his four weeks at Kernan, but now I will backtrack to describe his cognitive progress while he was there. I had assumed that getting better meant everything would get better, evenly and smoothly. His mind would heal in parallel with his body. I didn't understand how different this was.

The Monday following John's admission to Kernan, seventeen days after the onset of his stroke, a speech language pathologist (SLP) evaluated him. The report of that encounter follows:

Listening: Unable to follow one step or simple directions without moderate to maximum cues, unreliable yes/no responses, no identification of objects to names given choice of two, severe expressive aphasia.

Reading: Did not test, no identification of numbers or letters given choice of two or three, does not recognize own name given choice of two.

Verbal: Able to state single words, unable to repeat, imitate or produce upon request, no naming, no functional language, some fluent spontaneous language void of content, severe expressive aphasia, volume soft and low.

Writing: Did not test, held pen but unable to form letters, numbers or copy stripes.

Behavior: Cooperative, good effort

Summary: Severe receptive and expressive aphasia, no functional communication, no evidence of understanding.

After reading the evaluation, I asked the SLP if John had global aphasia, a term I understood to mean "general" aphasia. The SLP confided that they didn't like to use the term global aphasia because it sounded so hopeless. (Actually, the term "global aphasia" didn't upset me. I'd never heard it before and so it had no negative connotation. Hopeless was the word I didn't like.) Instead they spoke of input, or receptive (processing auditory language, and reading) and output or expressive (speech and writing) abilities. The bottom line was that he couldn't understand what was said to him as evidenced by his inability to follow a simple instruction; his speech was void of content; and he couldn't read or write—not even his name.

He had a long way to go, and his recovery of language in the four weeks at Kernan did not mirror his physical recovery. John's hard work to recover physically was repaid with the return of movement and function in his right arm and leg. He steadily and markedly improved each day. His excellent physical condition prior to his stroke seemed to have helped significantly in his recovery.

Aphasia was a different ball game. Each day revealed simple things that he could not do. Stranger were the occasions when something that seemed much more complex to me was easy for him. Several times I witnessed bizarre behavior and wished I could understand it. As much as I wanted to help, I felt so unprepared for the strangeness of it all. It was as if John were living in a fog. Sometimes, some of the fog lifted and for a few seconds, he was John. He was normal. Then he slipped again back into the fog. Perhaps it was only my perception. As he began to recover physically, or when I would close my eyes and he would laugh or make an appropriate response, everything would feel normal for a few seconds and I would forget. Then he would utter a long string of gibberish or fail at what seemed such a simple task, and I would be jolted back to the present and remember again. Rescuing the mind was an enormous challenge. I didn't understand why John's high intellectual ability before his stroke didn't help his language recovery as much as his prior physical condition had aided his physical recovery.

As far as the prognosis for recovery, doctors and SLPs at Kernan were cautious. On the positive side, they expected some spontaneous recovery over the next few months as the blood drained from the hemorrhaged areas in his brain and the swelling subsided. They also predicted improvements as a result of his SLP sessions.

Predictions and case studies in books were so varied as to be useless, and they very rarely addressed patients whose strokes were caused by brain hemorrhages. With so little to go on, I felt an overwhelming need to believe that there was hope for, if not full recovery, at least great improvement. Perhaps we simply believe what we want to, given the slightest encouragement. One theory I clung to suggested that once the brain had physically recovered as much as it could, the patient's effort was the primary indicator of success. That was the only variable we could now control. I had to believe that John's recovery was, to a great extent, within our power to control.

At Kernan, John had eleven SLP sessions each week. He saw four different SLP therapists, two of whom co-shared a job, and different ones on Saturday. Perhaps that made it more difficult, but in any event, he seemed unable to learn anything they tried to teach him. They were all young, positive and friendly women. I shall refer to them collectively as the SLP. I usually sat to his right in the small office, where he could not see me or be distracted. I was there to learn and only rarely participated.

It started off simply. Three pictures were placed on a table in front of John, one of a spoon, a pencil and a hammer. He was given a spoon and asked to match the object to the picture. He had no idea what to do. The SLP demonstrated by placing the spoon on top of the picture of the spoon. Then she handed him a pencil and repeated the instruction. Still no clue. She placed the pencil on top of the picture of the pencil and handed him a hammer. He looked puzzled, not understanding what she wanted him to do. She completed the task and began again, laying out the three cards.

By the third time, John was doing the task correctly until she gave him the objects in a different order. Then it fell apart. He was not matching objects to pictures. Perhaps he was repeating a series of steps: the first object goes one place, the second object another and the third object still another. He seemed unable to grasp the concept that an object and a picture of that object were somehow related. Adding names (spoon, pencil, hammer) to them didn't seem to help. I later learned that there was a term for this inability to match objects to pictures of those objects—associative agnosia—so John must not have been the only person in the world who couldn't do it or it wouldn't have a name. But it seemed like such a simple thing to do. Why couldn't he do it?

He was unable to select an object from three, given the name. (Give me the pencil.) He was unable to correctly point to a picture from three, given the name. (Show me the picture of the pencil.) He could usually repeat the name of an object, but never two objects together and often he repeated instead the name of the last object, not the current one. If she said "pen", he said "pen"; then when she said "hammer", he said "pen" again. The last word was stuck in his head and he couldn't move on, a clear example of perseveration.

After a few days, there seemed to be little progress, but somehow I believed that John understood more than the tests revealed. I spent so much time talking to him each day and it seemed that he understood some of it. It just wasn't demonstrated by matching or pointing to or selecting objects. That evening on the computer, I constructed a page containing twelve blocks with clip art pictures of places John had been or activities he liked. Then I printed a duplicate page and cut them out. The next day, we experimented. I told him a story and asked him to match the picture to the story. It went something like this:

"John, remember when you went to Egypt with Shelly? You saw the pyramids and Sphinx. It was hot and dry and there was a lot of sand. You went inside a pyramid, down the dark tunnels into the tombs where the pharaohs had been buried. Do you see a picture that looks like a sphinx?" He correctly pointed to the picture of a sphinx.

"John, remember when you worked for NASA? You were responsible for a lot of different satellites. They had lots of different instruments on them and they circled the earth. One of these pictures is a satellite circling the earth. Do you see a picture of it?" Again he correctly identified it.

He continued to correctly identify people in a raft (from his trip rafting through the Grand Canyon), a man riding a bicycle (from his trips through Napa Valley), a man working in his office, a bar chart and a glass of wine, all with stories, but not a telephone, a cup or a file cabinet. Then he successfully matched the cut out pictures with the identical pictures on the single page.

So the single object didn't make sense to him, but he understood enough of the stories and seemed to remember his experiences. He could point to pictures that represented them. Single words, particularly nouns out of context, could just as easily have been spoken in a foreign language. They seemed to have no meaning. To understand, John needed a lot of context. As bizarre as this was, it didn't seem so terrible. The goal was to communicate. John needed to understand what was said to him. I never spoke in single words anyway, I tended to talk too much, not too little. I just had to keep it simple.

Janet, his occupational therapist, knew John had a mathematical background so she selected tasks that used money—pennies, nickels, dimes and quarters. The first week, she put a pile of change on the table beside him. On a sheet of paper, she wrote in a column 1¢, 5¢, 10¢, 25¢. Pointing to the change, and then to the 1¢, she asked him if he could find one. As always, at the start of the task, he didn't understand and Janet had to explain it again, and then demonstrate. She took a penny and put it beside the 1¢. Then she asked him to do it for the 5¢. He did, then found a dime to match the 10¢. John seemed to understand coins. What a joy to find some way he could demonstrate that something in his brain was functioning correctly. It had been nearly three weeks since his stroke and this was one of the first thinking tasks he seemed able to perform. Then he picked up a dime and put it beside the 25¢. My excitement quickly cooled. Janet was about to gently correct him, but he was completely focused on this task. He got another dime and put it beside the 25¢. Janet and I looked at each other and waited. He moved a nickel over. Two dimes and a nickel—well, that worked. We both laughed and praised him for his success.

So he could read numbers, recognize coins and do some addition. Outside of his therapy sessions, it became one of our games. He started with a big pile of change in front of him. I would write an amount on a piece of paper, maybe 47¢, and ask John to get it. He was able to calculate up to multiple dollar amounts—but only if I wrote down the amount, not if I just said it. Hearing the amount and seeing it written down, I was surprised to discover, involved two very different skills. Processing auditory data was apparently much more difficult for John.

Another day Janet handed him ten index cards with the numbers 1 to 10, written as numbers. He looked at them for a few minutes and began to sort them in order without being asked. So sorting made sense.

The SLP had given him cards with simple words and cards with corresponding pictures to match. The word "cat" on one card and a picture of a cat on another, a dog, a cup, etc. No luck. He could not match any of them. It appeared he could not read even the simplest nouns. Since he had successfully sorted numbers, I made up cards with the numbers written as words: one, two, three, etc. and handed them to him. Without being asked, he sorted them in ascending order. Well, he was reading something!

Next I made up index cards containing the names of the planets. Remember, this man's career had been with NASA. I wrote them from memory—all eight. I handed them to him and asked him if he could put them in order without telling him what they were. He looked through all the cards twice and looked up, puzzled. I was pressing my luck but it had been worth a try.

He said, "One?"

"One what, John?" I asked.

He pointed to the cards and said "one" again, this time with conviction.

I could only remember eight planets, but thought there were nine. Did he know that one was missing?

"John, is one missing?" I asked, laughing and feeling pretty stupid. He nodded and began to sort them. I wasn't sure about the order of the last three and didn't know which one was missing, so that was *my* homework that night! John was right. There are nine, and his ordering had been correct, except of course for Neptune which I had forgotten and he couldn't tell me.

How could he read and sort the planets, but not associate the word cat or dog with the picture of the animal? Did words make more sense than pictures or objects? Was sorting easier than matching? Did the planets fit together in some context? Were words like dog and cat lost but not Mercury, Venus, Earth and Mars? It was so puzzling, yet it was clear that he could read something. So I tried other words that John might be able to read in context.

John had always loved to travel. He had fond memories of many cities he had visited. Matching countries and cities would test both his reading and his memory. I made a set of ten cards, each with the name of a country that John had visited, and a corresponding set with the name of a city in that country. I placed the countries in a column on the left side of the table and gave John the cards containing the cities. He looked through both sets of cards, smiled and understood. This game was fun. He picked the ones that were easiest first, had to guess at a couple, and finally matched them all correctly, Rome to Italy, Madrid to Spain, London to England, Athens to Greece; and so on. He could apparently read all of them at least enough to know what they meant, in context, but he could not say any of them. And he still could not match a picture of a cat with the word cat. So bizarre.

John was unable to name anything around him. He couldn't say his name or mine or anyone else's, but over time, he knew whom I was talking about because he could point to them in pictures or imitate their behavior in a way that made us laugh. One of his funniest imitations was of his three-year-old grandson, Johnny. Since John Andrew and his family lived in Las Vegas, he had only seen Johnny a couple of times. I pointed to a picture of him, not sure he would remember. John laughed, produced his devilish grin and began to spit, shooting imaginary objects out of his mouth. The summer before, they had visited us in Maryland. Eating watermelon in our backyard, John Andrew had spit the seeds into the garden. Johnny had imitated his daddy, shooting both the seeds and the watermelon as far as he could. Perhaps spitting is not a great thing to encourage in a child, but we had all laughed at this little boy, trying so hard to be just like his daddy. John's memory was fine. So was his humor.

The SLP suggested we get a calendar and use it every day to orient him to the month, date, day of the week, and cross off the days as they ended to help him understand time. She gave him pages of blank clock faces with times written under each one and he correctly drew the hands on the clock. As it turned out, he understood time fine. We also used the calendar to talk about when people were coming to visit. Using a daily schedule taped to the armrest of his wheelchair and his watch, he always knew when he had to be somewhere, but didn't know where he had to be. The exception to this was mealtime when his wheelchair seemed to move on automatic pilot into the dining room.

John could repeat words of no more than one or two syllables, but not point to an object someone named, such as a door or a window. He could say the Lord's Prayer by rote and most of the words were recognizable until they became garbled near the end, but he couldn't pick up in the middle or repeat after me a single phrase in it. Part of automatic speech, a string of memorized words, they said. Automatic speech was fluent and spontaneous but devoid of content and not something he could control. Nevertheless, we said the Lord's Prayer a lot because it made both of us feel good to hear him speak so fluently and correctly.

Speech was emerging but it was mostly gibberish. His gestures and intonation were intact, but most of the sounds he made were not words. He seemed unaware of the fact that his speech was incomprehensible. Sometimes the words we thought he was trying to say had the same number of syllables as the sounds he made, but the resemblance ended there. It was not a consistent substitution of one sound for another. There was no consistency. His sentences were long and rambling, often twenty or thirty words, with perhaps only three or four words intelligible. Medically, the term was paraphasia, where all the sounds are jumbled and transposed, and it persisted throughout his stay at Kernan.

One day, his speech was taped. What follows is the transcription of John's response to the question, "Can you tell me a little bit about your family?" The jargon and stuttering are apparent.

> *"Ah, right for interioram, um, the the arterberant terbarate is, uh, belong of um us. This is actually going to be serbing because it doesn't boat delaps of those. Uh, uh, Kam, I is furz furziz, co, colachur, um, who's the the stameris of one who divicats that uh, our our security what I do and what what she does. She's she's, ron she's very good. She's excellent and uh, returns her— no, this, no, no, this is true. In terms, in terms of her her visage of what she could judge.*
>
> *"I think, the gemi eyes. Uh, it's been a long time, it's it's approxi about four, probably, presse pretty about four oddeseyums which was occurred to the odominate from the the the scourages, so its actually a false of four, geritise on the vask, and this this vask was where, that's uh, that's essential. I'd say that's it. It's, it's very,*

*it's foil to the the anaptuse for which I found in our youpanant jorge on that you
ask and I have no idea what's going to be convantee (laugh), but I'll try the best I
have."*

Gradually, as words emerged, automatic speech improved. Common
phrases, "in fact", "slowly but surely", "in terms of", "I have no idea", "Thank
you, I appreciate it" were spoken often. Numbers and adjectives were most
common. Pronouns were present, but often incorrect. John randomly
interchanged "he" and "she". Prepositions were placeholders, often in the right
place, usually the wrong word. Descriptive verbs were rare. There were three or
four generic and abstract nouns he used, words like data, system, and thing.
One day, every recognizable noun was "data", another day he might use the
word "system" to describe everything. Otherwise, there were few nouns that
made any sense. Wherever a noun belonged in his sentence, the sounds were
gibberish. Because his gestures and intonation were intact, and his speech was
not slurred, it was almost as if you were listening to someone speaking a
foreign language. If you could watch him on video and turn off the sound, he
would have seemed normal. John was not the least self-conscious about his
speech; he was oblivious. He had always enjoyed talking, and the fact that we
didn't seem to understand did not deter him.

Yes/no questions presented a big challenge. Throughout his stay at
Kernan his responses were highly unreliable and improved only marginally.
Also, rather than answer yes or no, he would often ramble, as if explaining all
the ramifications of the question in a foreign language which we could not
understand.

A simple dialog might begin with the SLP asking, "Are you a man?"

"Yes," John would reply.

"Are you a woman?"

"Yes."

"No, John, you are not a woman. I am a woman, Eileen (pointing to
me) is a woman. You are a man." Sometimes she would go into further
discussion, describe anatomical differences, give examples of other men and
women.

"Are you wearing pajamas?"

"Yes." He wasn't. I wondered if he knew what pajamas were. He never
wore them.

And so it would go. Twenty, maybe thirty questions. Answers were
random and often long strings of gibberish. The SLP would correct him. The
next day, she would repeat the questions. The answers were no better.

The questions got harder, more abstract.

"Do dogs bark?"

"No."

"Yes, they do, John, dogs do bark."

He shrugged. Did he think she was asking him if he heard dogs barking? Did he understand the word dog or bark? I began to believe that not only could John not answer the question, but he ready didn't care if dogs barked. He preferred just talking, heedless or unaware of the fact that his gibberish was incomprehensible. Little progress was ever made with yes/no questions at Kernan. I also observed that, in his four weeks there, I was the only family member ever to attend any patient's SLP session. I chose not to comment on it, satisfied that I was allowed to stay.

Every night a menu arrived in John's room for meals the next day. Initially, I filled them out. An SLP suggested that it would be a good activity for us to do together. He usually had three choices for each main course plus drinks, salads and desserts. We tried it. After an hour, I was ready to kill someone, John, myself or the SLP. John was incapable of making the simplest decision. "Do you want coffee, tea or milk?" was an impossible question to answer. Finally, I reworded the questions to ask him if he wanted something that I knew he liked, questions that required yes/no answers. It probably didn't work, but he seemed content with the food and it spared my sanity.

John often talked in numbers. They seemed to make sense to him. Weather was in degrees, activities were in terms of the time they occupied, and events he remembered might be in terms of the year they occurred. He might say, "It's about 54..." He was outside and referring to the temperature. It was not unusual for him to say, "There are four..."

"There are four what, John?" That was as far as he could get. We became good at charades, used lots of gestures and I racked my brain trying to figure out what he was talking about. Fortunately I had been a math major also. I could relate to numbers and tried hard to follow his thoughts. Amazingly, it often worked.

Just before he left Kernan, he had been running a fever. He was being monitored closely and understood that he would not be released until the fever subsided. Though no definitive cause was ever proven, when his medication was switched from Dilantin to Tegretol, his temperature returned to normal. He was with an SLP when two doctors stopped by to visit him. After a brief conversation, Dr. Makley told him his temperature was normal. John smiled pleasantly but didn't appear to understand. The SLP pointed to his head and wrote 98.6°. John looked pleased and said, "Ah, good." Thank God for numbers.

Throughout his stay, John was unable to follow verbal commands unless they were accompanied by gestures that were indicative of the action required. Upon entering her office, the SLP would say, "John, would you please close the door?"

"Okay," John would respond, but he did not move. She showed him the door. She closed the door. She explained what she wanted him to do. Next day. "John, would you close the door?" "Okay." Still, he made no attempt to close the door. Did he not understand the request, or was he unable to act on it?

He lost all words associated with body parts. He had no idea where his nose was, or his teeth, or ear, or any part of his body. We pointed to it, we said it, we wrote it, we used pictures that had labels for him to copy the words. He left Kernan still unable to name or point to a single body part. The SLP said it was not uncommon. I thought it was bizarre.

Prepositions were lost. He could not show the difference between under and over, in and on, in front of and behind, before and after. When he used prepositions in speech they were placeholders, but usually not the right placeholder, as if any preposition would do. "To" could mean "for" or "with", as in "Is it okay to you?" Odd that he knew he needed a preposition, but not which one.

By the time John's right arm was working again, we discovered that his signature was completely intact, although smaller than it had been. But he could not write a single word on his own. He could copy written letters, but could not write ones that were spoken to him. He would write the alphabet over and over again, copying each line from the line above, but he could not say any of the letters. Instead he might say the number that corresponded to its place in the alphabet, A was 1, B was 2, up to about F, before it got too difficult. He spent hours copying his name, address and phone number, but couldn't remember it or say it.

He could write numbers that were spoken to him with frequent "neighborhood" errors. He might write the spoken seven as 6, 7, or 8. He was correct about one third of the time, but was within the neighborhood almost always and could usually correct it with a second or third try. Usually, in order to say a number that was written, he had to count, starting at one, and stopping when he got to the correct number. Zero, obviously, presented a challenge.

He was unable to read anything aloud, but something about the written word was still there. Sometimes when he was struggling to say something and we were unable to communicate, he would use his index finger to write the first letter of the word on his palm. He usually did this with names of places, never common nouns or verbs. But he formed correct letters and they were usually the correct first letter of the word. My exercise was to guess whether "E" was England or Egypt, "I", Israel or Ireland? He usually acknowledged when I guessed correctly. It was not that he could spell, nor could he say the letter that he traced in his palm. It was as if he had a mental image of the first symbol that began the series of symbols that represented the word—but each symbol had no sound or name attached to it in his mind. It was more like the word was a picture composed of letters.

If aphasia is the name given to the damage to language functions, then there was also something else that impaired his perception or reasoning skills.

Eating, for example, was a confusing process for John. I stayed with him for most meals and he usually ate in the ward dining room. Utensils seemed to make little sense. One night, he tried to eat a bowl of tomato broth with a fork. I watch for a moment, waiting to see if he would realize his error. After several attempts, I handed him a spoon and said, "Try this, I think a spoon will be easier." He accepted the spoon and continued to eat, not seeming surprised or embarrassed. He tried to eat mashed potatoes with a knife, sliding the knife under the mashed potatoes and putting the knife in this mouth. I handed him a fork and suggested he use it. He accepted it without comment. Could you really lose a skill as basic as using the right utensils? I found this to be one of the most bizarre effects of his stroke. He knew what to do with a razor, a toothbrush, even dental floss, but not a spoon or a fork. That never ceased to amaze me and was a constant reminder of the strange things that must be going on inside his head.

I learned later that this strange behavior had a name—ideational apraxia, or conceptual apraxia. Apraxia refers to difficulty in carrying out purposeful movement like eating, that cannot be attributed to muscular weakness or lack of coordination. His problem was not that he could not hold a fork, but that his brain could not determine that he needed one. Apraxia occurs frequently in conjunction with aphasia and comes in many forms. For one person, it might mean difficulty in carrying out a simple movement, like waving good-bye. Another, when asked to show how to comb his hair might demonstrate by using his fingers as a comb, rather than showing how one would hold a comb. Still others might have difficulty with some complex sequential actions. In John's case, his apraxia problem manifest itself in his selection of the tools he needed to eat. I would later discover other tools that would confuse him, like when he tried to hammer a screw into the wall or dig a hole in the garden with a screw driver rather than a hand shovel.

John's recreational therapist, Sandy saw him twice a week. In a few sessions, we sang songs. Many childhood songs like "Row, row, row your boat," were part of his automatic speech and John could sing those with clearer words than his regular speech. He could play blackjack, still being able to add written numbers, and board games that required spinning a wheel or throwing dice and moving some number of spaces around a board.

Another activity, ping pong, turned out to be a minor disaster. As with most such events, it also provided a good learning experience. By his third week at Kernan, John was able to walk and use his arm well enough to attempt a recreational sport that involved physical movement, so Sandy took him into a room with a ping pong table. Since John had spent most of his time at Kernan in a wheelchair, his right field of view deficit hadn't been too observable. This activity made it glaringly obvious. The small, fast moving ball, flying across the table, disappeared just as it reached the center of John's pre-stroke vision. The table below disappeared from his field of view when he focused on the ball. With his weak right arm, he swung wildly and enthusiastically at the object he couldn't see, that moved faster than his eyes could track it, as he lurched out on his weak leg to hit it. Just as the ball disappeared, so too, the paddle he held was not visible to him, his hand was not visible, his leg was not visible. He banged his invisible paddle against the invisible table, and knocked both his invisible hand and his invisible leg against the edge of the table. It took less than a minute to realize that this wasn't to be his sport. Sandy stopped him immediately. Neither of us had realized the impact of this visual deficit, and fast movement compounded the problem. John was okay, but fast sports that required good hand-eye coordination were probably out. A ping pong table was one less investment to consider when John came home.

Another day, Sandy's project for John was to repot a plant. Sandy picked this project in the last week of his stay because John had enjoyed gardening before his stroke. For the task, she provided a pot, a bag of potting soil, a hand shovel, a watering can filled with water and a small plant from a local store. John appeared to understand the assignment. Then he picked up the watering can and began to pour water into the empty pot and watched as it spilled onto the table and floor. Again I wondered, what was he thinking? Was his sequencing screwed up?

In the four weeks John stayed at Kernan, he couldn't learn to use the nurse call button on the side of his bed, or for that matter, the radio, TV or bed adjustment buttons. Perhaps it had something to do with his eyesight, but I don't think so. In any event, he had to be strapped and locked in bed every night. He soon grew to hate it; a healthy sign, I thought. One night in the first or second week, I forgot to lock him in. He fell out of the bed that night and I was justifiably scolded by Cheryl. After that, he never balked about being locked in, but still could not learn to use the call button. Most nights, I would play a CD that he selected, crawl into bed with him, fully dressed minus shoes, and snuggle with him until he fell asleep. Then I would lock him in his bed and leave for the night. One time, forgetting something, I returned to the room to discover John still awake. If he was pretending to be asleep because I was tired, I would gratefully go along with his kind deceit.

In spite of John's garbled speech, he seemed to enjoy the visits of family and friends. His automatic speech was fairly good and he appeared to understand enough of what was going on, and recognized enough words to understand and respond. We used a lot of gestures and body language, and tried to keep things simple.

Kathleen, Mary and John's mom came down two weekends for a few days each. Their excitement and enthusiasm encouraged John as he showed off his new skills. Brendan and his wife Jeanne flew in from Dubuque for a long weekend. The last time Brendan had seen John, he was virtually unconscious, with a dismal prognosis. Being active in the Dubuque Catholic community, Brendan and Jeanne had asked local convents, monasteries and churches in Iowa to pray for his recovery. They believed it was working. Christopher visited from Salt Lake City for a few days. John's daughter, Janet, was there at least once a week. Annie and her husband Jeff came several times. My son, David, came home from school one weekend to see him. These visits, which he eagerly anticipated, were good for him and for his family. It would be hard to imagine a patient having a more supportive environment in which to recover.

When his daughter Janet came to visit him a few days after he arrived in Kernan, she asked him if he knew her.

"Well, of course I do," he responded.

When Jeff, Annie's husband asked him if he'd like a Guinness, he replied, "You betcha!"

To my explanation of what happened to him, his stroke and surgery, he said slowly, "I need to think about this."

So it wasn't all gibberish. But the fact that I documented those comments the day they were made, shows how remarkable I perceived them to be at the time—those brief moments of normalcy.

Except for family, Art was the only person John wanted to see. Initially when John arrived at Kernan, he struggled just to get through the day and visitors would have been too exhausting. As he stayed awake longer, I thought he would like to see his friends again. Many people had been asking about him and following his progress. One evening, he had two unexpected visitors, people he knew from work. They stopped by after we had finished dinner and John was already in bed. They were cheerful, and chatty, filling him in on the activities at work, and stayed about thirty minutes. John smiled when they smiled, laughed when they laughed and seemed to follow what they said. They kept telling him how well he looked, how much better he was than they expected him to be, how everyone at work was anxious for him to come back.

When they left, John's expression changed as he looked at me and said, "No more."

"You don't want them to come back?" I asked.

"No one."

"You don't want any more visitors? John, you have a lot of friends who want to see you."

"No one. None," he said angrily.

I started to disagree, to try and persuade him to see some of his friends, but he apparently felt very strongly about this. Perhaps he was embarrassed or found it too exhausting. Perhaps he felt like he was on display or thought he should have been able to entertain them. Perhaps he knew he would never go back to work, or maybe he was just totally lost by their conversation. Whatever his reason, he didn't want any more visitors. I learned from this that well intentioned people can create very upsetting situations. I knew that I would never again visit someone in the hospital unless I was sure they wanted visitors.

Why was recovery from aphasia so much slower and more difficult than his physical recovery? Was the blood receding from the areas in his brain that controlled his physical movement but not his communication skills? Was the damage there more severe and permanent? Was language so much more complex than movement?

Of course I cannot draw any medical or scientific conclusions. As his wife I could make observations, noting what worked and what didn't. As a regular observer, and occasional participant in his SLP sessions, I felt that the sessions were useful primarily to identify things that he could not do. He seemed incapable of relearning (as opposed to recovering) any of the communication skills he had lost, although he did improve somewhat during his stay there. I attribute the improvement to spontaneous recovery in his brain as the blood and swelling receded, and to the constant interactions he had with all the people around him, the nurses and therapists, his family and friends.

I spent seven to ten hours with him most days, usually from nine until noon, when I left for work, then from four until he fell asleep at night and all day on weekends. In the beginning, I don't think he understood even five percent of what was said to him, though that understanding increased with the use of body language, and visual clues. By the time he left Kernan, using a totally subjective and personal rating system, I believe he understood about twenty-five percent of spoken communication when given in context.

Interestingly, other people, especially his family and visitors, thought he understood most of what they said to him. Since they knew he had great difficulty speaking, they carried on the bulk of the conversation, looking for appropriate responses and simply agreeing with most of his gibberish. They perceived a language production problem, not a comprehension problem. I learned then how easily one can determine the appropriate response from the speaker's tone of voice, facial gestures and pauses. John was a master at reading body language and intonation. He could respond appropriately with "yes, yeah, really, wow, that's great," on cue, virtually every time. A frown from them would elicit a frown from him. They thought he understood everything and were astonished by his progress. From time to time I would test this theory, making a sad or bizarre statement in a cheerful tone of voice. His response usually matched the tone of voice, not the statement. Two months before, if he had been sitting at the kitchen table, hidden behind the morning paper, his response would have been irritating but normal. Now, as he sat focused and concentrating, it was neither. But it was improving and body language was important. The goal was to communicate.

John always lit up when I arrived in the morning, and later, after his nap, when I returned before dinner. Each afternoon, he would be sitting in his wheelchair, either in his room or by the nurses' station waiting for my arrival, eagerly checking out each new visitor. I never felt as special as John made me feel when I walked into his unit.

Though he was usually cheerful, he was also capable of feeling great sadness, usually directed toward the suffering or pain of others. He never seemed to feel sorry for himself and what had happened to him. Rather, he was very sad to see the condition of others in his ward. After two weeks, he acquired a roommate, a man about his age who also had a stroke. The man was frequently depressed and cried a lot, refusing to eat or actively participate in his therapy. John felt sad for him and the other patients. He would point, say it was so terrible, and look so pained. I sometimes wondered if he knew he was one of them.

During those weeks at Kernan, I felt a wide range of emotions, but not the ones I would have expected before this happened. In many ways John and I shared the same feelings, and that was fortunate, for we often reacted to each other's positive attitude. I learned that depression is a natural and normal reaction, a part of the recovery process for many stroke survivors. Everyone, doctors, family and friends, expected John to be depressed, but depression had not been a part of his makeup before the stroke and it did not surface now. I don't know why he never got depressed. Perhaps his brain damage somehow prevented it, or some chemicals in his brain kept him content and cheerful and motivated to get well. It may have been a characteristic of neglect, a disassociation of himself from what happened to him, but he just didn't seem that concerned. This odd contentment was much easier to live with than depression. Right or wrong, I was relieved and grateful.

Many stroke survivors and their loved ones view their life in terms of what they have lost. Instead of being one hundred percent, they are only ninety, or seventy or fifty percent. They begin to define themselves in terms of their limitations, in terms of what they can no longer do, and they naturally grieve for that loss. I had often looked at strangers and felt sorry for them because of their limitations. I would have expected myself to feel that way about John, about us. But I didn't.

Overnight, back in April, John had gone from one hundred percent to almost zero, but he was alive and each day there was progress. Maybe one percent, maybe more, sometimes less, but when measured against zero, it was always good. John wasn't coming from one hundred percent, he was coming back from zero, and during that time, we could both genuinely rejoice in his progress. Perhaps we had so much hope because his physical recovery was so remarkable. We expected the same improvements in his mind. Though he was often disappointed in his mental performance, as when he couldn't remember his address after copying it for an hour, it only seemed to make him more determined to do better. Instead of quitting, he always wanted to try again.

Sometimes when he felt embarrassed or discouraged, it was my turn to be the optimist, to find humor in the situation. "John, it's okay to make mistakes. You're supposed to make mistakes. It's safe to make mistakes here. In fact, when you stop making mistakes, they kick you out. Don't worry about it."

Shortly after the stroke, I believed that John was still there, lost somewhere inside his body, inside his brain, and the challenge was to bring him out again. Perhaps I was still in some sort of denial, but I truly never felt that John was diminished, rather that the whole John was still inside, somehow cut off, blocked, from the rest of us. His bridges to the outside world had been torn down and needed to be rebuilt. When I saw a devilish look in his eye, or felt his hug, or held his hand, or watched his pantomime to tell me a funny story, I knew he was there. I believed he could emerge again, and knew he wanted to.

The John that was emerging was a kinder, gentler John, a man who lit up when I entered the room, who constantly wanted to touch me, who held my hand and said he loved me. I was falling in love with this man, perhaps I realized, for the first time.

I felt such tremendous pride when I saw how hard he worked to recover. John was an inspiration to me. There was little room for sadness. It was exhausting, and exciting, and worrisome, and loving. We both shared the same determination to get better and we both completely believed he would. Hard work didn't scare either of us, rather it challenged us, and kept us from being sad.

Ten years earlier, I had started a training company. We were in the business of training adults and as a key part of that, I had often given speeches on the concept of the lifelong learner. I encouraged people to view life as a discovery process, a continual learning experience. Though I had never imagined how close to home it would hit, lifelong learning was just as valid for John now as for the rest of us. John and I both had a lot to learn and our life was far from over; it had just become incredibly challenging.

We were both dependent and vulnerable. I needed John as much as he needed me. We both wanted and needed him to be as independent as he could be. That was always our goal. We never lost sight of all the things that he could still do. As humans, we spend our whole life learning—we just can't know in advance what it is we'll have to learn. I had to believe that John could learn again. The concept of the life long learner took on a whole new dimension, and my philosophy a new conviction.

The human mind has such a strong need to communicate. When verbal skills are lost, the need to connect remains strong, and with both of us,

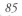

physical communication increased immeasurably. Our hands, our eyes, our faces, became the best tools we had and the barriers to our former relationship melted away.

I never knew how much better John could get, or how much better he would be tomorrow, or how long it would take until ... until what? Until he was better? What did that mean? Every day was better than the day before. There were no easy answers. I only knew how he was each day as we lived it, and I found I could accept that. Acceptance and resignation are not the same thing. Acceptance allows for hope, and we certainly had a lot of that. But I also knew each day, that if he never got any better than he was that day, it would be okay. Each day was to be lived fully, struggled through, enjoyed and shared. We were not alone; we were together.

10

A Business Decision

The weeks at Kernan flew by swiftly. Still operating in survival mode, I was handling the small decisions and the urgent ones, but the one that seemed too big I had parked on the shelf for another day. That day was fast approaching.

At issue was what I would do about *Fastrak Training Inc.*, my company. No, it was more than just my company, it was my baby. It was my love. It was my success and over the years, as my boys grew up and my marriage settled in, it came to define who I was. Through it, I was an entrepreneur, a business developer, a financial analyst, a professional speaker, and underlying it all, I was a teacher who loved to learn as much as to teach. After that, I was a mother, and finally, a wife.

In a more traditional time, in a more traditional woman, the role of wife, the duties and obligations, would have been more central, the decision perhaps simpler. But this was not that time, I was not that woman, and the decision before me felt enormous.

By John's third week at Kernan, it became clear that he would be coming home soon. John would need a full-time caretaker—24-hour supervision Dr. Makley said. Who would that be? Could I find someone, the right someone, to be with him all day while I worked, to stay all night when I traveled? Could I cut back on my hours, eliminate the travel, get part-time help and try to be both a caretaker and businesswoman? Or should I close the business and focus completely on John's recovery, perhaps getting consulting work occasionally?

I was a woman in a man's world, had been for a long time, but I believed that this was a decision few men would feel compelled to make. How many men would consider folding the business they loved to care for their wives? In my gut, I knew, had the tables been turned, John would have tried diligently to find a good caretaker for me, but would not have considered closing a business to do it himself. But this wasn't John's problem and how he would have solved it, though niggling in the back of my mind, was not relevant. This was my problem, my decision, and the decision I made had to be one I could live with. I felt secure in knowing that decisions I'd made in the past had turned out well. What was far less certain was what I wanted to do now.

The second oldest of seven children, I was born to an Irish-German Catholic father from the Bronx, and a southern-Baptist mother from Georgia who converted to Catholicism because in the early 1940's, if you wanted to marry a Catholic, that's what you did. My parents had grown up during the depression and instilled in their children a strong work ethic and a sense of responsibility and duty. Mom cooked and cleaned, chauffeured us everywhere and was the empathetic, non-judgmental role model who simply believed that you did whatever had to be done. She raised us to believe that we could accomplish anything we set our minds to. Whatever happened, we could handle it, nothing was impossible. She dealt with life's aberrations calmly. "It's not the end of the world," she would say. And with each of our successes, "I knew you could do it."

Pop worked at General Foods, and rose through the ranks, retiring as the Controller of Bird's Eye in 1974. When he wasn't "working" working, he was helping the church with their finances, or running the little league. He was honest and ethical, a good man, father, and neighbor. I remember the cold Sunday morning, returning from church with all nine of us piled in the station wagon, when pop spotted a man whose car had ditched in a snow bank. He pulled over long enough to tell the stranger he'd be right back. After taking us home, he returned with a shovel to help the man dig out. Pop's life was work, family, church and community. He was unquestionably my white knight. In my world, mothers always loved you. Fathers could be proud of you. My foremost goal, through much of my life, was to make sure he would always be proud of me. In my private moments, I imagined myself to be my father's oldest son with all the connotation that carried, though Richard would later claim that title. It wasn't my birthright, but I was determined to earn it.

By most standards, I succeeded. I attended sixteen years of Catholic schools, including an all girls' high school and a woman's college. I came to believe in later years that the all-female schooling provided opportunities that a coed environment in the 1960's could not have. Competing against boys, and at the same time wanting to be popular, might have limited my achievements. Girls weren't supposed to be smarter than boys, but at Immaculate Heart Academy I found a circle of friends who were smart and competitive and we excelled together, though they all graduated with higher GPAs than I. Some years the boys I dated were boyfriends, some years, buddies, but the only intellectual male competitor I remember was the tall, lanky, red-headed date who was too uncomfortable to dance at the Bergen Catholic social. With a perfect 800 on his math SATs, we spent the evening sitting out the dances, challenging each other with math problems scribbled on the paper tablecloth in front of us. He felt comfortable in the world of math, and my mid-700 score, though good by most measures was no threat to this shy genius. We both enjoyed a game well played. Friends returned to the table to tease us, but I suspect we had more fun than most that evening. Back then, boys were expected to lead in school, but given the opportunity in an all girls' high school, I became president of the student council. At Dunbarton College, long hours of study paid off when I graduated at the top of my class with a degree in Mathematics.

With a mother who believed I could accomplish anything, schools that provided the opportunity to lead and excel, and a father who was proud of me, I developed the self-confidence I would need in later years to start my own company.

Directly out of college, I had worked as a contractor on projects related to the space program and the defense and aerospace industry. Over the years, I had been a programmer, a software engineer, and later a software manager. I understood the complexities of software.

In 1987, my boys were entering adolescence. Until then, my job had afforded time to be a soccer and baseball mom, a den mother. Now David and Sean spent more time with their friends, less at home. I was ready for a new challenge.

The seeds of entrepreneurship were planted when a friend from work invited me to go into business with him. He, John and I, and a third man would provide the capital; I would run the company. His idea was novel, ahead of its time and would require a lot of concept selling before it could succeed. We explored the idea for months but I discovered that, while I loved to read about pioneers, I was not one of them. I would be more successful selling something for which the world perceived a need, rather than persuading the world that there was a need for what I was selling. Although the idea was discarded, the seed grew and the excitement of entrepreneurship took hold. I felt the glass ceiling that prevented women from intruding too far into the male dominated engineering fields in the 80's. I was a software manager on a project that would take years to complete, and I was bored.

I chose the business of training for two reasons. First, I loved to teach. Even as a young child, in second or third grade, I would gather up all the "little kids" and play school. I was, of course, the teacher. In high school and college, I tutored. As an adult, I assumed the role of teacher whenever the opportunity presented itself and it often did. I can't deny that I loved an audience, loved being in front of the class, but there was also real satisfaction in watching someone learn, in seeing light bulbs go on in their heads. There was excitement in a sudden look of discovery or understanding in their eyes. I knew I could teach people about software.

The male perception was my second reason. I had encountered enough men who were threatened by female managers. I knew that in order to succeed in a field dominated by men, my business could not be perceived as threatening. I also knew that every little boy grew up with a female teacher in front of the classroom, and for the most part, accepted it as a natural part of their universe. Females as teachers were not threatening in the same way that females as bosses were. Training, in the business world, was a support role, but could be a very influential one. "Leading from behind" I called it, and was secure enough to find it amusing. And so, at the age of 39, I founded *Fastrak Training Inc.*

Like most new entrepreneurs, I expected to be rich in a few years. My original, very naive business plan made it seem so easy on paper. But the first three years were unbelievably hard. We lost money while I worked long, long hours and then lay awake at night trying to figure out how to pay my employees. The only thing worse than the worrying and the eighty-hour weeks was the fear of failure. Giving up was not something I could bring myself to do. I always wanted to give it a few more months.

I loved *Fastrak*, but I never anticipated how all consuming it would become, how it would spill over into every facet of my life, how focused I would become on its success. I also learned that teenage boys, regardless of how much time they spend with their friends, need a lot more attention than I gave them in those years. So do husbands.

Initially, John was incredibly supportive, even providing much of the startup money. But over time, seeing the problems I faced and how difficult and consuming it was, both personally and financially, he wanted me to close up shop. I was always tired and worried and my business had clearly become a source of tension between us. Sex, when we had it, was brief and distracted. Fights over the cleanliness of the house were resolved with a maid service every two weeks. Dinners were usually late, quick, and rarely memorable. Reluctantly in 1991, I agreed to give it just one more month, awaiting the announcement of a big long-delayed competitive procurement. We won the contract and everything turned around. That success led to others and within three years we were listed in INC. magazine as one of the 500 fastest growing, privately owned companies in America. For two consecutive years, Washington Technology magazine identified us as one of the 50 fastest growing high technology companies in the Washington DC area. Our clients, initially drawn from the military and federal government and their contractors, grew to include a strong commercial segment and eventually many of the Fortune 500 companies.

Payroll was no longer a juggling act. I could pay myself, and repaid John's loans with interest. We became recognized in our niche industry of training software professionals. That recognition led to public speaking opportunities in which I promoted the need for training in our industry and life-long learning among our professionals. Life-long learning became a favorite topic of mine.

Now I was at a crossroads. John could not be left alone. Despite his remarkable physical improvement, he still hadn't walked more than a few feet. His cognitive and language skills were progressing slowly. There was no way to predict how much better he would get. This man couldn't learn how to use a nurse call button after three weeks of explanations and demonstrations. His speech was mostly jargon. His vision was impaired and when he walked, he constantly bumped into things. He only understood a small part of what was said to him. He had trouble determining what utensil to eat with. His thinking was often fuzzy. He couldn't dial a telephone, and even if he could, he probably couldn't ask for help—if he knew he needed it. I had no idea what he might do with an oven or a stove. He couldn't be home alone now and there was no way to know if that would ever change.

I considered three options. The first—employ a full-time caretaker. I explored this option with John's caseworker at Kernan. She gave me a list of agencies that provided this service. John didn't need a nurse. He needed someone to be there for his safety, someone who would drive him to daily therapy sessions, someone who would talk to him, be a companion, help him regain his lost skills. Even if I cut back on my travel and worked only eight hour days, John would still be spending a lot of time with this person. At about $150 a day, that would cost about $37,500 a year and insurance didn't cover it. And there was still the cost of therapy. I didn't know how long he would need outpatient therapy or how long our insurance would pay for it.

His caseworker warned me that a caretaker is basically that. The job entailed keeping him safe, not all the other things I wanted. It was often a low-skilled and low paying job, with most of the money going to the service agency. Caretakers were generally not trained to provide the range of services that I wanted for John and high turnover was common in the field. Even if we found someone wonderful, he or she could leave in a few weeks. I didn't believe that John would ever be able to return to work, not with all the limitations he had. What if John recovered enough that he no longer needed a caretaker? Would he be alone all day? What would he do every day by himself? There were adult "day care" centers. The thought of John spending his days there depressed me. I would worry and feel guilty all the time. What about the quality of his life? I investigated the possibility of hiring college students, or grad students who were studying speech pathology. I called some schools, but the results were not promising and time was running out.

The second option—divide my time between work and John. Stop traveling. Hire instructors to cover the training that I was doing. Perhaps turn over some of the management responsibility to someone else so I could spend more time at home. But I liked training and running the company. If I wasn't managing and I wasn't training, what would I be doing? The caretaker problems would still be there, but to a lesser extent. Hiring good instructors was always difficult and the uncertainty of the company's future had exacerbated the problem. Two strong prospects that I had interviewed before John's stroke had declined job offers in the last three weeks.

This was the solution that most people recommended, the middle road. It allowed me to buy time, to see how John improved, to delay making a major life decision with everything else that was going on. But to me, it was deciding not to decide. I was already exhausted a good deal of the time. I had lost ten pounds since John's stroke. Those first ten pounds delighted me, satisfying my perennial new year's resolution, but at the rate I was losing weight, I risked getting sick. That was something we couldn't afford right now. I was already feeling guilty that I had been neglecting work. This option seemed to insure that I would feel guilty about leaving John when I was at work and guilty about work when I was with John. Would I ever have a spare moment to myself? I was afraid this option would consume me and leave me feeling like a failure—doing nothing well. Fear of failure had always been my biggest fear.

Finally, I could close the business to be with John full time. This was the most permanent option. If this was my decision, it probably couldn't be undone. From a business perspective, even the work that was involved in closing the business was daunting and there were employees to think about. Most would have no difficulty finding new jobs. They would have offers as soon as the word got out. For the administrative staff, it would be more difficult, but the economy was good and I could help them.

If I wasn't working, would we have enough money for the rest of our lives? Money always scared me—having enough that is. I had no pension. We lived comfortably, but not extravagantly. I doubt I owned anything that hadn't been bought on sale and our evening meals usually reflected the grocery specials that week. Vacations always found us at AAA discounted motels. Our home was large and comfortable, but the custom drapes were made from fabric that I scavenged from an old warehouse in Florida at 75% off. I put a large premium on value. In the last several years, our "peak earning years" as the experts call them, after paying for David and Sean's college, I had saved every cent I could, investing in mutual funds and bonds. I knew John had his own investments, but I didn't know much about them. We kept our money separate, except for common bills. So I needed to understand where we stood financially.

Fortunately, a few months before, we had both begun to organize our investments on our computers—he on his, me on mine. I had money in several

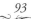

different places. So, I learned, did John. Since I was in saving not spending mode, I hadn't been paying much attention to it as an aggregate. I didn't know how much John had. I hadn't thought it any of my business then—it was his money, not mine—but now it was important. Establishing the collective value of stocks, bonds and mutual funds was tedious but straightforward, requiring a search of both computer and paper files to organize it in a single spreadsheet. The company where John worked, NYMA, was about to be sold, and John had stock options, but it was too soon to tell how much that would add or what taxes would leave of it. I had never put a value on the assets of _Fastrak_ beyond the tangible real property which was small. Training was a service not a product, so it hadn't seemed useful to assign a value to our courseware. After talking with several people in our industry, I concluded that licensing the courseware was probably the best way to generate additional money. Thank God the '90s had been a good time to be socking everything into the stock market. The amount we had surprised me.

Working with yet another spreadsheet, I projected our income, which included John's pension from NASA, disability income that he would receive until he became 65, and our income from investments. I might have future consulting income, but needed to know if we could live without it. I calculated our expenses, knowing that the mortgage was almost paid, and set aside a generous sum for medical costs, believing that was now the biggest unknown expense. There were some big unknowns—John's stock options, my future income, medical expenses—but unless the market took a long, serious dive, I decided we would be okay. The decision didn't have to be made on financial grounds. In one sense it was a big relief; on the other hand, it meant that the need for income could not be the excuse for keeping _Fastrak_ open.

But spreadsheets couldn't answer the hardest questions. Could I give up my company for John? How would I spend all the hours in all the days for the rest of my life? I was 48 years old. Until the stroke, John and I had led very full, independent, and busy lives. Given our jobs, and all our travel, we had averaged about an hour or two a day of our waking time together over the last twelve years, and there had been times when that seemed like too much. What would it be like to be together 24 hours a day, forever? Would we be okay if he never got any better, or just a little better? What if he recovered completely? Would I resent him? I couldn't blame him for what had happened. I didn't blame him. But committing to spend all our time together forever was awfully scary and seemed so permanent.

I pondered the answers for hours. Nights, after I left John sleeping at Kernan, I lay awake in bed, not knowing what to do. It felt as if I were being asked to choose between a husband and a child—so unfair. Before John's stroke, I'd received more positive feedback through _Fastrak_, than I had from John. My company had come to define me. Who was I without it?

In the last few weeks, so much had changed. John had changed—physically, cognitively and emotionally. It was his emotional changes that now drew me to him. We had both spent years not being vulnerable to each other. Before John's stroke, we both seemed to view vulnerability as a flaw, pride as the shield that protected us from getting too close, from risking pain. Seeing how fragile life was, how quickly it could be taken away, we now knew how vulnerable we were. With this unspoken acknowledgment, long-standing barriers disappeared. Finally, after all these years, he needed me and wanted me and loved me. I didn't remember ever feeling that John needed me before, but after the trauma of the stroke, I knew that I needed and wanted him. I wanted him to recover and didn't believe that anyone could help him as much as I could. What surprised me most was the discovery of how much I loved him. I couldn't explain it. I just knew it was true. A powerful tug-of-war was pulling me apart. I kept looking for a fourth option. But the decision had to be made, and it wasn't one that could be decided with the toss of a coin.

In the past, John was my sounding board for major business decisions. I respected and valued his opinion, even when I didn't follow his advice. We did talk about this. It was a warm spring afternoon and I wheeled him outside to sit in the sunshine. I described the options I saw, having difficulty separating the logical from the emotional. John understood that I was considering closing *Fastrak*, and we both understood that only I could decide. His life had already been profoundly changed by a bizarre twist of fate. Should I, could I, choose to give up that which had come to define me? He looked as sad as I felt. He knew how important *Fastrak* was to me. During his stay at Kernan, it was the only topic that ever brought tears to his eyes. Mine too.

Since all the options were viable, in the end, I had to decide based on how I felt about it. Whatever decision I made, I knew it would be the best I could do at the time. I did a lot of soul searching and some praying. What should I do?

One night, alone in bed pondering the future, I discovered one simple truth. In the five weeks since the stroke, when I was with John, I never wished I was at work, at *Fastrak*. When I was at *Fastrak*, I always wished I was with John. Spreadsheets aside, I had already made the decision. I had fallen in love with this new man, and that surprising discovery would close another chapter in my life and start us on a new journey.

I wasn't afraid. Certainly there was sadness, and more tears would be shed in the future over the decision. But they were the same kind of tears that I shed when I graduated from high school and college, when I left the company where I had worked for almost fifteen years to found *Fastrak*. The tears were an honest tribute to a wonderful adventure, to friendships that would probably end, to life lessons learned; a normal, healthy way of putting the past behind and moving on in my journey through life. I felt peaceful, restless and excited.

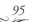

Peaceful in the knowledge that it was the right decision. Restless in that, once the decision was made, I wanted it to happen quickly. Excited at the prospect of truly sharing life with my new husband, of being the vehicle for his recovery. It was the hardest decision, it was the easiest decision. I couldn't think of a single thing I'd rather do at this juncture in my life.

At the office Monday morning, May 19, four days before John was scheduled to come home, I called everyone into the conference room. I told them what my options were and how each option would affect them. I thanked them sincerely for all their support. Then I announced that I would be closing the office by the end of the summer. They understood. It was a sad day. We hugged and cried.

Odd how, when all is said and done, it usually comes down to some simple truth. I had made the only decision I could live with.

After three weeks at Kernan, John was well enough to count down the last seven days until he would come home. It was late May. After a cool spring, it was finally warm outside. John didn't like being confined to the wheelchair. He didn't like being strapped and locked in bed at night. He didn't like being shut indoors in the afternoon, waiting in his room or at the nurses' station for me to arrive. He wasn't crazy about the food anymore. (So much for the idea of macaroni and cheese when he got home!) He wanted to be outside in his garden. He wanted to sleep in his own bed. He wanted out. I thought these were good signs. He was recovering.

When the fever he had been running the last week subsided the day before John was to be released, we were relieved and excited. It was his last barrier to coming home.

Annie's husband Jeff installed a new stair railing. I didn't know if we would be bringing a wheelchair home with us. At Kernan, he was always in his wheelchair except during physical therapy sessions. Would he need a wheelchair when we went to the store or a restaurant? Susan's answer made a lot of sense, "He can walk until he gets tired, and then he can sit down and rest. A wheelchair is more likely to be in the way."

As it turned out, endurance was not the problem. His vision was. Because of his field of view cut, John often didn't see things on this right side when he walked. He was more likely to bump his leg or bang his hand against something than he was to get tired. He had to train himself to scan as he walked and we usually held hands or walked arm-in-arm wherever we went outside the house. It was one of the plusses of his stroke. We were physically closer and both liked it that way. Another plus was that one of his few perfect sentences was "I love you," and he said it a dozen times a day. The doctor claimed it was automatic speech. It struck me as odd that, coming from John,

"I love you" could be considered automatic speech, judging from the few times he had said it in the previous twelve years. But who cared? I was more than willing to say it back, or say it first.

Preparations were made to the house before his return. David was home now and he nailed wooden 2x4s around the perimeter of the low parts of the deck so John would feel them and not fall off the edge. We removed rugs in heavy traffic areas. I purchased a shower chair and an inexpensive hand-held shower spray. Since he could walk, most of the obstacles I had anticipated were no longer problems.

The week before he left Kernan, he got a haircut from a volunteer barber who came once a week and charged $2 for his services. The kind man, faced with a big challenge of stubble where John's scalp had been shaved for surgery and long thinning hair everywhere else wasn't a miracle worker. John's $2. haircut at Kernan wasn't much of an improvement over his $50,000 "haircut" at Maimonides. I had been able to overlook my teen age boys shaved heads and ponytails. At least John's haircut was not an act of defiance, and it would grow.

The day before he left Kernan, John weighed 150 pounds. He had lost 20 pounds in six weeks and looked fragile. He had a minor residual weakness on the right side of his face, and his eyes often looked dull, glazed. Sometimes they were John's eyes, and they sparkled, but that was the exception. The dullness in his eyes was the most vivid physical reminder of all that he had lost. I hoped that, in time, as he got stronger, they would regain their alertness. His eyes truly seemed to be a window into his soul, capturing the shock of what his body had done to him.

When the day finally arrived, I could barely contain my excitement. I remembered my earliest visions of John coming home, just after his stroke when I had imagined him sleeping on a bed in the den, hooked up to oxygen and a feeding tube, me sitting beside him holding his hand, hoping he would wake up, not knowing if he would recognize me. Instead, I was returning with this wonderful man who knew and loved me, who could walk and laugh, who wanted to touch me and hold my hand all the time, who was motivated to get well, who was happy and still had a great sense of humor. We were so lucky. I couldn't believe my good fortune. There was life after stroke and we were filled with hope.

Together we packed up the items in his hospital room. There were over a hundred get well cards from friends who thought of him and prayed for his recovery. We met with Dr. Makley for John's final debriefing and received his prescription for Tegretol, instructions for his care, discharge papers and an appointment to return for a follow-up visit in two weeks. I had debated asking him the "big question" for a couple of days, but my need to know overcame my cowardice. With a fair amount of awkwardness and eyes averted, assuring

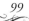

myself that no one was within ear shot, I quietly asked Dr. Makley if John could have sex. What must he think of me? John had just had a "catastrophic" stroke, and I'm asking about sex. Dr. Makley handled my embarrassment in a matter of fact way. He said that there was nothing to prevent it. There was no reason why John couldn't have sex if he wanted to. Life was getting more normal by the minute!

May 23, 1997 was a beautiful warm spring day. We walked around the TBI unit, saying our good-byes with heartfelt thanks. We now counted several of the nurses and therapists as our friends. We loaded up the car, put the convertible top down and drove away. It had been exactly six weeks since John's stroke. This was his first taste of freedom. Baseball cap firmly in place, he put his head back, breathed in deeply and grinned from ear to ear. He was going home.

John observed his surroundings as I drove. Within a few minutes, he seemed to know where he was. As we approached the turnoff for my sister's house, he pointed to it, saying, "There's your ... brother's..."

"You mean Annie's house?" The term "brother" could mean any relative.

He nodded. A few weeks ago, I wasn't sure he had any concept of what home was, much less where it was, and now he was correctly showing me where other people live. His brain struggled with so many things. It was always a wonderful surprise to discover something that was intact. His sense of direction was one of those things. John knew exactly where he was, and over the coming weeks, though he might confuse the words left and right, by pointing he gave directions that were perfectly correct.

Sean came home from Albuquerque for a couple of weeks. I was delighted by John's progress, but Sean had seen the John of one hundred percent, not the John of zero. Even though Sean and I had talked on the phone about John's condition, he couldn't have been prepared for the different man he saw now. It made Sean very sad, and at first his reaction surprised me. Then it forced me to realize how other people who knew him before his stroke would perceive him. Most of John's speech was jargon. His comprehension was low. At twenty pounds lighter, he looked frail. John had come a long way in six weeks, but perhaps I was the only one who saw him through rose-colored glasses.

We were arriving home the Friday before Memorial Day, giving us three whole days together before I had to think about work again. I watched John closely, afraid he might have a headache or his fever would return. I was afraid he might do something to hurt himself, afraid he might get confused, afraid I might do something wrong that could be dangerous. I was afraid to let him out of my sight. It was important to get things back to normal, but I just wasn't sure what normal meant now.

In the "olden days", I cooked, and John cleaned up the kitchen, loaded and unloaded the dishwasher, cleaned the counters. That seemed like a good place to start. Unloading the dishwasher turned out to be the most challenging of these tasks. Silverware was confusing. We still had his and hers silverware from our prior single lives, kept in different kitchen drawers. Sorting it took him a long time, but we had time, and I left him alone to do it. He often didn't know where some item went, odd bowls, cups, all the miscellaneous items in a kitchen. Naming the items was no help. Kitchen items were lost somewhere in his head and difficult to retrieve. Was this a "guy" thing, I wondered?

Laundry presented no problem. He had always done his own; I did mine. He wanted me to check that he was doing it correctly, and he was. He selected his own clothes to wear each day but wanted confirmation that his choices were okay. Usually they were except he tended to overdress for the weather. Having lost 20 pounds, he now felt chilly more often. Actually, this had a positive side effect. Before, I had always been the cold one. Many a "car fight" had erupted over control of the temperature settings. Finally our body temperatures matched. Now we both had cold feet in bed!

John remembered which nights the garbage went out, and which days they collected the recycled materials. That was better than I could do. So far, so good.

Showers were a challenge for a couple of weeks. Afraid he would slip, I insisted that he use the shower chair and the hand-held spray. Since our shower was actually a standard size tub with a sliding acrylic door, there wasn't room for John, me and a shower chair inside, and everything got wet when the door was left open. After several bathroom-soaking showers, I finally relented and let him stand up alone in the shower. I stood outside the door, prepared to rescue him if need be. Again, he was fine.

I anticipated our first sexual encounter nervously. I certainly didn't want him to have a heart attack or another stroke. Should I take it slowly or try to get it over with quickly? Sex wasn't something we typically discussed and with the unreliability of his yes/no answers, asking him was unlikely to produce a legitimate response. Our unspoken signal in the past had been for one of us to close the bedroom door and see how the other responded. I waited until he had been home a few days. Then one night after he had washed up, brushed his teeth and gotten into bed, I looked at him and closed the bedroom door. He grinned. Memory was okay. By the time I hopped into bed, it was apparent that body parts were functioning properly too. We both laughed. John wasn't wasting much time. Since John's stroke, we were physically closer and much more affectionate than we had been for years, and it was apparent that night. I needn't have worried. It was physically and emotionally satisfying for both of us and not something I would worry about again. It felt good to be alive.

There was one thing that bothered me. I know it's an ego thing, and it embarrasses me to admit it, but it's true. John couldn't say my name.

Occasionally, he called me Kathleen, his sister's name. Sometimes Janet, his daughter's name. Usually, if he called me anything though, it was mom. Of course, he couldn't help it, I knew that. It was automatic speech. They were names he'd said as a child, or young man, names he'd said long before he met me, but it still bothered me. I didn't want to be his sister, or his daughter, and I certainly didn't want to be his mother. I even asked my boys when they were around him, to call me Eileen instead of mom. It was a difficult word for him to pronounce, as were all words that started with a vowel sound, and though we practiced it for a while, it seemed just too difficult for him to remember or to pronounce. There were so many other more important things to work on, that eventually I gave up. It seemed egotistical to focus on it, but in moments of frustration, I wondered where he had been the last twelve years. It bothered me that my name wasn't part of his automatic speech.

The Monday following his release from Kernan, John began his outpatient rehabilitation at Horizon, a clinic about ten miles from our house. During his initial evaluation, the PT decided that he would not require physical therapy. His gait was steady and smooth. Because his arm and hand were still weak, the OT suggested exercises that he could do at home, but formal occupational therapy was not necessary. He had come so far!

In contrast, language testing indicated little improvement from his initial evaluation at Kernan except now he was much more alert and would try to respond. In the area of auditory comprehension, he was still unable to answer yes/no questions, or follow commands. In verbal expression, he was unable to name any of thirty common objects, or complete any of ten sentences. He could repeat twelve of one hundred words. In the "jargon" of the SLP, *"Utterances were characterized by fluent jargon, multiple neologisms, perseveration ... patient appeared unaware of his erred responses."* Reading comprehension was the most promising, showing he could match written words to common objects in a field of two with eighty percent accuracy, verbs with sixty percent accuracy. He could sign his name, copy letters, words and sentences, but not write letters of the alphabet to dictation, nor write words spontaneously. The overall impression was "severe receptive and expressive aphasia of the fluent type." He clearly needed language therapy, and we established a daily schedule for these sessions which we would both attend.

The three months following John's return home were incredibly hectic and full. Having made the decision to close the business, I had much to do at work. By the end of the summer I needed to make as much money as possible licensing our courseware, knowing that once the employees were gone, I wouldn't focus on marketing *Fastrak* anymore. The employees were wonderful as hundreds of letters were sent to clients, explaining the situation and offering licenses for courses we had taught. Course materials were packaged with lesson plans, course descriptions, electronic and paper slides and sample textbooks.

Thanks in a large part to Beth's hard work, the response from clients was overwhelming as most elected to obtain the packages and we worked frantically to prepare and ship the material. I also needed to close up the office with its 4000 square feet filled with furniture, computers, books and office supplies; resolve the lease; help employees find new jobs; and continue to meet all the training commitments we had already made for the summer. My son David worked part-time for *Fastrak* that summer and stayed with John in the afternoons while I was at the office.

Since John could be easily confused by changes in schedule, we established a routine for our days. Each morning began with a drive to his SLP sessions. With few exceptions, I attended those sessions and participated. During the drive, he would practice speaking, warming up for his meeting with the SLP. He would practice saying the days of the week, months of the year, counting, and saying the alphabet. If he began with the days of the week, it was impossible for him to transition to the months of the year alone. The days of the week were still in his head, and he couldn't get them out to say something different. This was true regardless of what we started with.

It was as if there was room for one sequence, but then it was stuck there, and wouldn't go away to make room for the next. Perseveration was a significant problem. Usually, I had to get him started (January, February, ...) or he didn't know which sequence I wanted. He seemed to know that the words day, week, month and year related to time, but knowing which one started with Monday and which one started with January was beyond his ability. The beginning of a sequence was better than the end. By the time he got to "September" in the sequence of months, it was pretty garbled. Counting was the easiest for John, but he couldn't remember when to stop. We also said the Lord's Prayer. He seemed to feel more confident with these morning warm-ups.

The forty-five minute SLP sessions were similar to the ones at Kernan with yes/no questions, repetitions, naming objects or activities, and completing phrases. He usually had homework to complete for the following day.

After his SLP sessions we would drive to my office. The employees at *Fastrak* were kind and patient with John. I would work for a couple of hours while John would do some of his homework, and then try to play solitaire on a computer. In the beginning he was incredibly slow and missed most of the moves. I had never realized how complex solitaire is. You have to be able to count. On the bottom, the cards go from high to low, on the top from low to high. On the bottom, the colors alternate, on the top, they must be the same suite. You click to turn over cards, and move them using the mouse.

This was far too complex to explain to John and it seemed beyond him, but I was busy. He understood that I had to work, and he seemed content to try. After four weeks of trying, John won his first game. He came running in

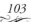

to drag me to the computer. Everyone in the office came to see and congratulate him. When I suggested that he play again, he said, "No more, I won." He had met the challenge and it was no longer important to him. He hasn't played solitaire since that day.

Usually in the afternoons, if I had to work, David would drive John home. After his nap, John and David would go for a walk in the neighborhood. John would work in the yard, occasionally watch television, and try to read some of his magazines. I hated being in the office when John was home, but there was so much work to do. Having made the decision, I looked forward to closing the office.

David and John had never been close and I worried about their time together. In the past, it hadn't taken long before they got on each other's nerves. A look, a phrase, a tone of voice would easily set the other off, and could quickly escalate into a shouting match or slammed doors. Now they interacted very differently. David was amazingly patient with John, listening and trying to understand him, explaining things that John couldn't understand, repeating things he couldn't remember, taking long walks with him. Each day when I arrived home, John said David was great. David, responding to John's praise, tried hard to be a good companion. David was a big help that summer. I couldn't have managed without him.

There was one business trip I had to make in June. Months before, I had committed to teach a four day course in California, and couldn't, in conscience, renege. Kathleen and John's mom drove down for the week to stay at our house. His brother Brendan, with his wife Jeanne flew in for a couple of days. I didn't ask them to come, but I probably couldn't have stopped them if I wanted when they found out I had to leave town. I truly did appreciate it and John was happy they were there. David, I suspect, was a little overwhelmed. My sister Annie took time off from work and planned activities for them. She knew John loved bonsai and scheduled a trip to the National Arboretum. Another day she drove them to the zoo. Annie marveled at John's ability to direct them. She had a general idea how to get there. John knew the best way to go, even where to park.

Although John had not wanted visitors other than family at the hospital, he seemed ready to start seeing a few friends again. Art and his wife Cinda were his first visitors. I was pleased to have guests, wanting John to stay in contact with the world as much as possible. John was happy to see them. Art was his usual outgoing, casual, friendly self. Cinda hadn't seen John since the stroke and couldn't know what to expect.

To me and to Art, John was making so much progress. Cinda compared him to the John she knew. Her face revealed far more than her cheerful conversation conveyed. Poker wouldn't have been her game. She couldn't conceal the incredible sympathy she felt. I was reminded of Sean's reaction—the recognition of how much he had lost, not the vision of how far he had come. I wondered if I had made a mistake by not letting John's friends see him sooner. It was important that she understood how I felt so I spoke to her before they left.

"Cinda, you look so sad. Please don't feel sorry for John. He's come so far in the last two months and he gets better every day. Our life has certainly changed and I know this sounds crazy, but in a lot of ways, it's better than it was before. John's a wonderful inspiration. Things aren't bad, just different. We'll both be fine. Look how happy he is. Just give him time."

I knew she would come to understand it and believe me over time, but I also knew that it was hard right now. Over time, she did understand. In the coming months she became one of the many people who marveled at how wonderful John was. They left with Art promising to call and get together to "hang out" soon.

Roger, a friend of John's from his Goddard days, had sent several cards and personal notes while John was hospitalized. He and I had spoken on the phone while John was at Kernan. He had listened to my early tales of how disabled John was and had very low expectations when he came over shortly after John returned home. Roger was amazed at the extent of John's recovery.

Roger was the man who had hopped an airplane with John to visit Iceland one weekend in the dead of winter after I had quickly rejected his insane invitation. The remote possibility of seeing the aurora borealis was easily offset by my dislike of frigid temperatures. So I thought they were both crazy. Roger and John could go several weeks without talking, and then, upon meeting again, could pick up the conversation as if no time had elapsed. I had a couple of friends like that and valued those relationships.

The visit was delightful. Roger and I talked, John listened and occasionally joined in. Roger and John made plans to have lunch together soon. I insisted that they go without me. Though Roger made it clear that I was welcome, he didn't seem to feel uncomfortable being alone with John. It was important to me that John maintain a part of his life that was separate from me, and Roger, like Art, had my full endorsement. When he left John felt great. Naturally, so did I.

Richard and Barbara were one of the few couples that John and I both liked and saw frequently. A few years earlier, the four of us had gone on a cruise to Alaska. They had wanted to visit John at Kernan, but respecting John's wishes, I had asked them not to come. A few days after John's return home they invited us over for dinner. They were good friends, fun to be with and very supportive of John's recovery. It was important to me that people didn't feel uncomfortable around John, and they were great. John and Richard had been friends since their early Goddard days and John seemed comfortable talking to them even when he didn't make much sense. They took it in stride

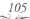

and encouraged him to participate, without embarrassing him. It was to be the first of many evenings spent with these close friends who helped us deal with our challenging times.

The Kemper Open was in early June. Every year, Pete, the president of NYMA, and his wife Cathy held a big party at their house on the golf course, and we had always gone. This was John's first outing with many of his friends from NYMA and Goddard. I was excited and nervous. John was mostly nervous. Everyone seemed sincerely glad to see him. Knowing that he had been paralyzed by his stroke, they were amazed by his physical recovery. I stayed by his side and responded to questions for him that required more than a simple acknowledgment. His ability to read their body language and respond appropriately to acknowledge understanding, caused most of them to believe that he understood much more of what they said than he actually did. Everyone came over to say how wonderful he looked, how much better he was than they expected, how much he understood. John received their congratulations saying, "Thank you, I appreciate it." It was a good phrase to be able to say. After about two hours he was exhausted and we left, but he felt satisfied that they hadn't understood the full extent of his disabilities. That seemed important to him.

July 6 was my mother's eightieth birthday. A surprise party was organized in Atlanta at my sister Katherine's house. It was to be a big family reunion and I wanted to go, but was worried about John traveling. The doctor said it was okay for him to fly. Annie and Jeff were flying down with us. Richard hadn't seen John since the day after surgery, Paul a week later. The rest of my family, mom and pop, Katherine, Mike and Dorothy had been in touch frequently by phone, but hadn't seen John since his stroke. John had always been a favored spouse, well liked by everyone in my family, a "good catch", as I was often reminded. Everyone was anxious to see him again.

Packing, the night before, took a long time. I wanted John to select what he would need for the trip. Thinking it through was difficult for him. Remembering to bring enough socks and underwear for several days, and the right clothes for different events was confusing, but it was important to let him try, and he did. After an hour we went through his choices together, made some changes, added a few items, and packed his suitcase. Everything we did took much more time but we had time. I was learning patience. So was John.

Checking in at Baltimore, I discovered that the airline had switched our seat assignments on the leg from Charlotte to Atlanta. We were no longer seated together and they couldn't change it in Baltimore. We could try to change our seats in Charlotte. Our flight was late arriving in Charlotte; the airport was crowded; the line was long; the flight was overbooked and boarding. There was no way I would let John sit alone. He couldn't request a drink, or say a complete sentence to anyone. If he had a problem, he would need help. I anticipated a battle as I watched disgruntled passengers turned away at the counter. The protective lioness instinct was surfacing. My adrenaline was flowing, my mind preparing what I would say, not wanting to cry or to scream. Finally, facing the agent at the counter, the panic clear in my voice, I handed him the boarding passes and blurted out, "We have to sit together. My husband's had a stroke. He has aphasia. He doesn't understand what people say and when he speaks, he doesn't make sense. He can't be alone."

I had no intention of getting on that plane unless we were seated together and I was prepared to be as confrontational as necessary. The agent looked at me, a woman clearly on the edge of hysteria, then at John, calmly oblivious to my ranting, punched a few numbers in his computer, and handed us two boarding passes with adjacent seats.

"Oh. Oh, thank you." As relieved as I was, it was almost anti-climactic. No battle? Now I had to calm down, to let the panic subside.

In Atlanta we rented a car. Annie and Jeff rented another one. They were going to stop and eat along the way. Did we want to join them? Since I rarely ate breakfast or lunch, the timing of those meals was something I left up to John, and hungry was a word John knew. It amazed me how much he could eat.

"John, Annie and Jeff are going to eat now. Are you hungry?" I asked.
"No."

"It will take about an hour to get to Katherine's house. If you want to eat, we should do it now. Do you want to eat?"
"No."

So we got into our rental car and headed for my sister's house. Less than thirty minutes passed before John announced he was hungry. I had to keep reminding myself that John's yes/no answers were still very unreliable. I spend my life being in a hurry. I always want to get "there", wherever "there" is, and this time was no different. I wanted to get to Katherine's house. I didn't want to ask for food as soon as we arrived. When John was hungry, as he almost always was these days, his window of tolerance was narrow. I had two choices: I could strangle him or I could feed him. I decided that I'd invested too much effort in John in the last three months to kill him now, so I opted to make a fast-food stop. Patience—I still had a lot to learn about patience.

We stopped at a Taco Bell along the way. At least now John was willing to eat fast food. While I waited in line to order, John needed to use the bathroom. I pointed him in the direction of the restroom. Almost sixty seconds elapsed before I realized that he might not know which was the men's room. I rushed over. He was in the ladies' room—alone, fortunately. There were so many things to remember. I added one more to the list—make sure he knows *exactly* where the men's room is.

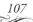

My family is large, loud, quick, funny and always on the go. During the next three days, Katherine's house was filled with people, my parents, my brothers and sisters, their spouses, and several small children. It was in this chaotic environment that I began to understand John's "filtering" problem, as I came to call it.

The best way I can describe it is through analogy. Imagine you're listening to an orchestra and you need to block out everything except the piano, or a violin—any single instrument. Then imagine that each instrument is playing a different song, so it all just sounds like noise. What tune is the piano playing, or one violin? For John, that is how I imagine it was when he tried to listen to one person in a room full of people talking. All the sounds were going into his head at the same time but the filter was broken. As difficult as it was to understand one person, speaking alone, it was impossible to filter out one voice from a crowd and then try to understand it.

At least for now John was alone in a group—lost in a cacophony of sounds that were as garbled to him as his speech was to me. We couldn't always avoid crowds, but as much as possible, we tried to limit most conversations to one-on-one. My sister Dorothy went with John for long walks, something they both enjoyed more than I did. John needed to be around other people without me, but he also needed to be safe. Dorothy, among others, fit the bill. They seemed comfortable together—and to be honest, I wanted to sneak away for a couple of hours to enjoy my favorite recreational sport—outlet shopping. I needed some time alone, not much, just a few hours, and I knew that a Saks Off 5th was less than twenty minutes away. It was my first separation from John not caused by work and the urge was too strong to resist.

My family's reaction to John and me was interesting. Interesting is the word you use when you don't really mean good and you don't really mean bad. They were relieved, pleased, worried, guarded, concerned, comfortable, uncomfortable, happy, sad, afraid, optimistic, and pessimistic. Several times I bragged about how wonderful John was, about how much he had already recovered, about how lucky we were. I meant it and really believed that he would continue getting better. We were doing fine. Everyone was very supportive, but some dwelt more on the enormity of the task ahead of us, as they witnessed John's frail state, his confusion at simple tasks, his inability to follow conversations and his incomprehensible speech. While I could not imagine failure, having seen so much progress already, they remembered the John of one hundred percent. They knew I was closing the business I loved. They worried for John, but perhaps even more for me. So much was unspoken, so much meaning imbued in simple phrases spoken so directly, "you take care of yourself now", and "call if you need anything". But I felt so incredibly strong and happy. I didn't see the problems. I didn't understand why they were so worried. But I loved my family and it was good to know they loved me too. And I thank God for my rose-colored glasses.

A week later we drove down to Kitty Hawk, North Carolina to spend a few days with John Andrew and his family, and Janet and her boys at the beach. We decided to stay in a motel rather than in the house they had rented—too many people, too many grandchildren, too difficult to filter, too exhausting. John Andrew hadn't seen his father since Maimonides and now enjoyed every moment with him. This visit was so much better than his last. I don't think John Andrew could have imagined during those long hospital hours as he sat beside his father, holding his hand, stroking his arm, telling him it would be okay, that three months later he would be standing beside him in the ocean surf, laughing with him as the waves pounded them both. John was unsteady, and John Andrew watched him like a hawk, but they were fine. I couldn't have imagined it either. They were wonderful moments for all of us.

There were two major breakthroughs that weekend. First, I learned that I was now be living with a back-seat driver. With few words and a lot of gestures, I found myself being told which lane to drive in, which cars I should pass, which gear I should be in, what the car temperature should be, and how fast I should drive. In the past John had usually driven when we were in the car together. This was a new experience for me. A year earlier he would have been walking on the side of the road, thumb extended, long before I reached Kitty Hawk given his level of "constructive criticism". Now, rather than being annoyed, I found myself amused. John must be getting better—this must be part of recovery. He had been a faster and more aggressive driver than I was. Sometimes I complied with his requests. Sometimes I laughed at him. Once I reminded him that patience was a virtue that we both had in short supply, and this time around, it was one we were going to have to learn. We both took it in good humor. My, how things had changed!

The second breakthrough occurred at the swimming pool of our motel. After suiting up, gathering the things we needed from our room, John checking and rechecking everything several times, me assuring and reassuring him we had everything we needed, finally, thirty minutes later we parked ourselves in lounge chairs. John then decided that he wanted one more thing from the room. I didn't feel like going back up to get it, patience still being a far from perfected virtue of mine. John indicated he would go. Could he find his way back to the elevator? Could he press the button for the correct floor? Could he find the right room? Could he use the key to open the correct lock of the two on the door? Could he find what he wanted and repeat the process in reverse? There was only one elevator. Our room was near the elevator on the second floor. The key had the room number on it. John and I had done it several times together. I knew he needed some degree of freedom and independence. His good sense of direction and ability to read numbers were in his favor. His inability to understand single commands, much less follow a sequence of steps, worked against him. I acquiesced. I reviewed with him all the steps he had to follow. Off he went. How long should I wait before going out to search for him? Less than two minutes passed before I was no longer able to read my book. Five minutes, seven minutes passed. He should have been back by now. I got up to go towards the elevator, afraid I'd made a mistake. Out he walked, successfully completing his mission, looking quite proud of himself. I was flooded with relief. This was his first adventure into the world alone since his stroke. Eight long minutes of independence.

Over the summer much of John's jargon disappeared. It was so gradual that it went almost unnoticed. Perhaps the biggest factor was that he became more aware of it and tried either to correct it or looked to others for correction. Unfortunately, the jargon was not replaced with content words, rather with more automatic phrases, strung together, that rambled on with no clear subject, no verbs and seemingly no periods. Most afternoons, when I returned from the office, we would sit outside and practice the names of common objects. Sometimes he had no idea what a word meant, other times his difficulty was in pronouncing it.

We played these games in the car and found it a good way to pass the time as we drove and it distracted him from his favorite pursuit—back-seat driving.

"John, can you show me a tree?" He couldn't. I would point some out. "Can you show me a truck?"

"A truck?" "A truck?" He would repeat the word, listening to the sound of it, thinking about what it might mean. He might point to one, or he might shrug and shake his head. Sometimes, he would know it. Other times, perhaps only a few moments later, he would not.

I would try dozens of words—car, grass, streetlight, stop sign, gas station, mailbox—each time we went driving. Most days he got some of them, different ones different times. As a concession to the advertising age, I must admit with irony, that he was more likely to correctly identify McDonalds or Mobil than he was to correctly point to a car or a tree.

Recovering from aphasia was like playing a probability game. For a normal, unimpaired person, learning a word means that you know it every time you hear it. If you know what a car is and I ask you to point to a car ten times in a day, you will succeed ten times. If you had aphasia, today you might be able to point to a car three times and not the other seven. Tomorrow, maybe more, the next day, perhaps less. The goal was not to "learn" the word "car", but to increase the probability of being able to retrieve the word when you heard it. The word "car" was not lost, the bridge to access and retrieve it was damaged—like a loose wire. The goal was to strengthen the connections.

A more important goal was to not get discouraged or frustrated. This was sometimes the harder goal to achieve. How could he identify it ten minutes ago and not know it now? I readily confess to moments of frustration, many moments, but when giving up is not an option, you simply keep trying. And so we did.

John loved to walk and began to take walks in the neighborhood alone. As with each new first (and second, and third), I worried, frequently looking out the window, waiting for his return. I didn't worry so much about him getting lost anymore. Usually I worried that something could happen to him and he couldn't get help. He always returned fine. My worrying was the price for his freedom and independence—a tough but necessary tradeoff.

By mid-summer, he wanted to start running again. We were both worried that it might jar his brain where his surgery had been, or that he might fall, not seeing obstacles in his way. The doctor said he could do it if he felt like it. That seemed to be the answer to most things—let him try. By fall, John was jogging two miles every other morning and feeling good afterwards. I was waiting anxiously for him to get home.

His friend Art came by occasionally, taking him out to lunch, and then going on afternoon adventures, one day sailing, another day to Gettysburg. Roger also came over and they would go out to lunch. John enjoyed these excursions. They were such an important part of returning to a normal life. (I later learned from Roger that after I had bragged to him about John running two miles, John confessed at lunch that it was actually three miles, but he didn't want to worry me!)

After John's release from Kernan, Dr. Makley directed us to another doctor, Marian LaMonte, who would continue to see John as an outpatient. She was the Neurological Program Director of the Maryland Brain Attack Center, an assistant professor of neurology at the University of Maryland Medical Center and a stroke specialist. She was tall, slim, attractive, energetic and positive. Dr. LaMonte believed that stroke recovery was an ongoing process and that stroke survivors could continue to improve forever. Motivation was a key factor in recovery. We found this very encouraging and chose to believe her.

She was amazed by John's physical recovery and intrigued by the marked contrast with his limited recovery from aphasia. She was impressed by his positive attitude and his motivation to improve. In an attempt to determine the actual cause of John's stroke and the likelihood of a recurrence, which greatly concerned me, she ordered a series of medical tests. Unfortunately, while the tests ruled out causes, they did not find any. Over time, the most positive result of all the tests was that Dr. LaMonte thought it unlikely that John would have another stroke.

By midsummer, I was mired in paperwork. There were medical insurance forms, disability forms, social security forms, doctor's forms—

everybody wanted medical history, among other things. There were ten-page forms, fifteen-page forms, forms that asked the same question over and over in different ways. There were forms that seemed totally irrelevant but had to be filled out anyway. Nobody could use anybody else's forms. All of the information had to be on their forms and many of them needed a doctor's signature. I kept copies of everything so that when forms were lost, I could resend them. We had survived the stroke. There were times I wasn't sure I would survive the paperwork. Being sick probably killed more trees than it did people.

John had contributed to disability insurance at NYMA. If the private insurance company determined that he was disabled, he was entitled to disability benefits. As long as he was classified disabled, until he was 65 years old, John would receive a monthly check. I had enough doctor's reports to document his disability. It was just a matter of filling out the paperwork. The private disability insurance forms were straightforward. I filled out John's parts, got the doctors to complete theirs, and NYMA provided the insurer with the work-related information they required. By September, two months after his vacation and sick leave ran out, they agreed that he was entitled to disability payments.

Applying for disability insurance from the Social Security Administration was far more complicated. The private disability insurance carrier required it because whatever Social Security paid would be offset by a reduction in the amount they paid. Though it reduced their liability, we wouldn't get any additional money.

After John was on Social Security disability for two years, he would be eligible to receive Medicare. Since he was no longer working, we were allowed by law to continue with the medical insurance we now had at NYMA until then, as long as we paid the full premiums. I knew that it would either be impossible or exorbitantly expensive for John to obtain other medical insurance in the future. I needed to be sure that he would qualify for Medicare when his current insurance expired.

Though Medicare was paid by the federal government, claims were investigated and authorized by the state, so the programs were integrated. The application and approval process took four months, pages of forms, dozens of messages left on answering machines and unreturned phone calls, misunderstandings, and crossed signals. At one point, they scheduled a psychiatric evaluation to measure the extent of his amnesia. I called to tell them he had aphasia, not amnesia. They promised to cancel the appointment. Two days later, the mailman delivered a summons to meet with the psychiatrist to evaluate his amnesia, scheduling the appointment in three days, when we would be out of town. The summons threatened to reject his application if he did not appear. Answering machines constantly intercepted my calls to both the agency and the psychiatrist. When human beings actually answered phone calls, they would try to straighten out earlier mistakes. I began to believe that it would never be resolved and found it thought provoking that applying for disability coverage could be impossible for a disabled person. Finally, he was declared "legally" disabled, though I never would have imagined that to be a victory!

Medical bills and insurance statements seemed to arrive daily. Organizing it all into notebooks was time consuming but necessary; understanding it sometimes impossible.

During the summer, John and I had been participating in his daily SLP sessions. In July, John had changed speech therapists again. Allison, a young woman just out of school, was now seeing John five days a week. She was enthusiastic and supportive and we hoped that she would be working with John for a while. We were extremely fortunate that John's insurance covered these sessions and all felt that John was making progress, but it was extremely slow.

As the end of summer approached, my life was getting frantic. By August 29, all my employees had terminated. David had returned to college. My landlord at *Fastrak* found a new tenant who wanted to move into our space in October. I was alone in the office with John in September sorting through papers, selling office furniture, donating supplies and equipment to the high school my boys had attended, and moving everything else into my basement.

John's brother Brendan and his wife Jeanne had invited John to visit them in Dubuque. John wanted to go. Although I was terrified at the idea of John flying alone, we scheduled it for the last week in September. It was the only way I could work fifteen-hour days to finish everything that needed to be done. I would join him at the end of the visit and we would fly back together.

John would fly directly from Baltimore to Chicago. Brendan and Jeanne would meet him at the airport in Chicago, and together they would drive the three hours back to Dubuque. After explaining the situation, the airline assured me he would be okay. Jeanne and I arranged multiple backup plans in case anything went wrong. I would call their neighbor when his plane left. They would call the neighbor to confirm lift off. They would call the neighbor when he arrived. The neighbor would call me when "my eagle had landed". Jeanne would call when they arrived home. These were the days before most people had cell phones and it appeared that telephone calls would cost more than the airfare. What if the plane had a problem and couldn't land in Chicago? What if traffic was heavy and Brendan and Jeanne were late? What if John got off the airplane and missed them? What if...what if...?

The airline let me board with John and make sure he was okay. The attendant promised to keep an eye on him. What if he needed to use the bathroom? Would he know to lock the door? I cried when he left. I was scared and exhausted. So many things could go wrong.

Even as I cried, I had to laugh at myself. My sister Annie had cried when each of her children started kindergarten, worried for their safety. Not only had I never shed a tear when my boys started school, I had rejoiced at their growing independence and my growing freedom. I had laughed at her foolish sentiment. Now I stood crying at the airport as my husband left to spend a week with his brother. A good lesson in empathy.

Everything went according to plan. The first night there, the archbishop of Dubuque stopped over to meet John and see how he was doing. Another day, they visited a convent where the nuns were anxious to meet the man they had been praying for. Later that week, there was a trip to the monastery where the priests and brothers had been praying for John's recovery. One of Brendan's clients was the Archdiocese of Dubuque, and Jeanne was an active volunteer in church activities, but I was nevertheless impressed. Brendan and Jeanne had enlisted the heavyweights to pray for John.

September drew to a close. Somehow, I managed to be out of the office by the evening of the last possible day. Nightly phone calls to Dubuque, though challenging, indicated that John was having a fine time. When I spoke to Jeanne the night before I flew in, she told me that John had a surprise for me when I arrived.

Packing my bags the night before, I remembered the handkerchief Brendan had offered me that awful night back in Brooklyn. I had washed and ironed it—probably the only time in my life I ironed a handkerchief. Now it was time to return it.

My flight was uneventful. I drove a rental car to Dubuque, arriving just before dinnertime and rang the doorbell. John and Jeanne approached the door together. Just as I was about to throw my arms around John, so glad to see him, Jeanne said, "Wait!"

I stood still. John looked at me and said, "Hi...Eileen." Jeanne had spent the week working with John, teaching him, among other things, to say my name. I hugged John, so proud of his effort. Then I hugged Jeanne and cried, overwhelmed by her understanding. She was now my friend forever, and my husband could finally say my name.

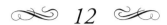

12

Our New Job

Perhaps it was the German blood from my father's side, but I never expected to stop working. Life was work. Closing the offices at *Fastrak* was simply a transition to a new job—one that John and I would share as partners, perhaps for the rest of our lives. Our new job was John's rehabilitation, and I undertook it with the same enthusiasm that I had for every new job. Although we had already been putting great effort into John's recovery, now we could focus on it without all the distractions of my business.

It was the beginning of October 1997. Almost six months had elapsed since John's stroke. With the *Fastrak* offices finally closed, the basement at home would be my new workspace. There was still a lot of work to do, organizing the basement, resolving the office inventory for record keeping and tax purposes, paying bills, returning telephone calls and doing occasional work for clients. But it would be on my time now, and I felt incredible relief at not having to worry about *Fastrak* every day.

Now it was time for us and we wanted to have fun. We had all day, every day, to spend as we chose. It was time to do the things we wanted to do. We had learned the unpredictability of life, and were determined to take advantage of each day that we had. The events of the last six months had brought us much closer to our families and we wanted to continue that.

One Saturday afternoon in October, Annie, Jeff and their daughter Darcy came over for a cookout. They arrived carrying badminton racquets and a birdie, and Annie announced that she wanted to play badminton before dinner. John shook his head and said, "I can't see it." I reminded Annie that because of John's visual field of view cut, he would lose the birdie in mid-air, and not be able to track it. It would be impossible for him to return a serve. I thought Annie might be a little embarrassed and apologize, but without missing a beat, she looked at John and said, "Good, he's on the other team!" A quick reminder of how deeply the competitive spirit runs in my family! We all laughed and John disappeared into the garage. He seemed to have taken it in good stride, but I hoped his feeling weren't hurt. Less than five minutes later he emerged. A badminton racquet angled out from each of his rear shorts pockets, another poked out from the hole in the back of his baseball cap. He held a racquet in each hand—making five in all, looked at Annie with a devilish grin and announced with a dare, "Now I'm ready." He looked so ridiculous, and was willing to make fun of himself. He could obviously hold his own with family and friends. John got a lot of respect and admiration, but he didn't seem to want or need or expect coddling.

Weekly tests during his SLP sessions indicated that his comprehension was improving, based on tests that measured correct yes/no answers, and following simple commands (raise your hand, close your eyes). His repetition was a little better. His ability to finish phrases was improved (salt and…, the cow jumped over the…), though often mispronounced. Silent reading indicated that he could usually select the correct picture for a simple sentence given two choices. Now that I was home full time, we could devote more time to his recovery and I hoped that he would progress faster.

Although we both felt that the time spent with Allison was useful, John now wanted to cut back his formal SLP sessions to three times a week. We weren't sure how long the insurance would continue to pay and thought that cutting back might extend the coverage period.

Since we would now be spending virtually all of our time together, it was essential that we establish goals. I had learned, many times in fact, from my experience training adults, that goals must come from the person who wants to learn, not the one who is going to teach. Most people think that the teacher should establish the goals since that is the way it is done in school and the teacher presumably knows what the student has to learn. In school, the curriculum is set, the child is taught and tested, and then promoted (in theory) when the subjects are satisfactorily learned.

This approach, often not particularly successful with children, fails miserably with adults. The goal must be important to the person who tries to achieve it, otherwise the motivation is either lacking or unsustainable, even with the most cooperative and willing person.

John had four major communication deficits that affected our lives daily. While his comprehension was gradually improving, it was still very low by normal standards. The more context he had, the more likely he was to understand. If a topic changed, he usually missed the transition, unless he was specifically made aware of it. If he was asked to point to his eyes, or his mouth, or his tongue, he would repeat the word several times as if searching for the meaning. He might put his hands near his face and say, "It's somewhere around here." Yet when he was told to close his eyes, or stick out his tongue, or shut his mouth, he could usually, but not always, do it.

His speech was poor, lacking content words, filled with badly constructed, rambling, and incomplete, but fluent sentences. He was more aware of his jargon, usually knew what he wanted to say, and would occasionally draw a picture to show an object. He usually acknowledged the word if someone provided it and would try to repeat it, but not always. Sometimes, he said that the supplied word was not the word he meant. We would try other words, only to discover after several failed attempts that the original word had it fact been the one he wanted. His gestures, which were completely intact, supplemented speech and made communication somewhat easier. He was almost never able to name an object given a picture of it.

Silent reading of single words, or short, simple sentences was haphazard—sometimes he recognized a word, most often proper nouns, or understood the sentence, other times he didn't. Again, context was important. But he could usually pick out the correct spelling of a short word, given three choices. Reading out loud was impossible—he was unable to say a word that he saw in print. The connections that linked the visual image of a word to the formation of the sounds necessary to say it were severely damaged. Words that he could say automatically and spontaneously were mispronounced when he saw them in print, even when he knew the word—as if they became twisted somehow in his head before they reached his mouth.

Finally, writing was the most damaged faculty. He could often print the first letter of proper names, but was rarely correct with other letters, although he often knew how many letters were in the word. If I said the word "king" and he knew what it meant at that moment, he might say, "There are four." Four letters, he meant.

When he tried to write a word, it was as if he was searching in his brain for the image of the letters. It appeared to have little to do with the sounds associated with the letters. He couldn't write anything from the way it sounded. He could sign his name. He could write, in script, Goddard Space Flight Center sometimes. If he got stuck, he had to start from the beginning, the way I have to do it if I'm repeating my social security number—the whole thing or the beginning, but not starting in the middle. And he couldn't print it. It was as if the few words he could write in script, came from his hand, not from his brain. Printed words had to travel through his brain and it seemed as if he were retrieving the picture of what the letters looked like. The sounds of the letters, whether I said them or he said them, did not help.

John and I spent a long time talking about what was important to him, about what his priorities were. John wanted to be able to talk to people, to say what he wanted to say. And he wanted to be able to read. He decided that writing wasn't as important to him as reading. He didn't seem to think that comprehension was a big issue. Actually, I don't think he understood how much he didn't understand. Telling him wouldn't help him understand it. We decided that in our time together we would focus on speech and reading. We agreed to put writing aside for a while. I came to the conclusion that he would actually be working on comprehension every hour of every day in order to function, so I wasn't too concerned. The goals he established were important to him, so they were important to me.

The big question was determining how to achieve his goals. I reviewed all the material John had been using in the last six months in his speech therapy. Since John's goals related to functional communication, it seemed to me that practicing repetition wasn't particularly useful. He needed to be able to express a thought that he initiated or respond to a question. If he was repeating what I said, then I already knew it, and it didn't help him with word finding, a big problem for him. Yes/no questions related to comprehension, not speech, but being able to name objects seemed useful and necessary.

While John had been visiting in Dubuque, Jeanne had purchased a box of children's flashcards. There were 96 cards, each with a picture of an object and the word beside it. If John could look at the card and name what he saw, I didn't know if he would be naming an object or reading a word, but they were both goals, so we added them to our communication tool box.

We'd both been building up frequent flyer miles for ten years without having time to use them. Now we had the time. John and I decided to take a three-week trip to the southwest in October, including a stop in Albuquerque to visit Sean. As we planned the trip, John remembered places that he wanted to see again. He couldn't tell me but he could read the AAA tour book well enough to recognize and copy the names of places he wanted to visit, and in a couple of cases, hotels where he wanted to stay. I made a chart which listed the date in the first column. John's job was to use the map and tour book to copy the name of the city he wanted to visit that day in the second column and the hotel, if he cared, in the third. We worked together to finalize the itinerary. I made the reservations. I'm not a good wanderer. I need to know where I'm sleeping at night before I can enjoy the day. John was less convinced of the need for this, but didn't mind going along with my wishes.

I was the driver. He continued in his role of driving critic. In many ways it was like a honeymoon as we often walked hand-in-hand, or arm-in-arm, and kissed frequently in public places. We were asked more than once if we were newlyweds. In some ways, I guess we were. It was so much easier to communicate physically than with words, but words sometimes provided the most amusing and memorable wrinkles.

One evening after dinner, we stopped at a drug store to buy postcards that John wanted to mail to his family. Next we stopped at a gas station to fill the tank. While John was pumping gas, I noticed the cards sitting on the front seat and put them in the glove compartment. I paid the attendant, received a ten dollar bill in change, and handed it to John as he closed the passenger side door. With my attention on the car, I turned on the lights and started the engine.

"Where is it?" he asked, as he began looking for something.

I assumed he had dropped the ten dollar bill and began looking for it. I didn't see it on the floor. I got out of the car and looked for it on the ground. There was no wind but it was nowhere in sight. It had to be somewhere in the car. I pulled over to the side of the station and we both began tearing the car apart.

"John, it has to be here somewhere. It can't just disappear. I gave it to you. Did you drop it?"

"No, I don't have it," he insisted.

We kept searching. I kept insisting that ten dollars couldn't just disappear as we began searching in the most impossible places. Several minutes later, as if my words were just sinking in, John gave me the most puzzling look and said, "Ten dollars?"

"John, I gave you ten dollars. Where can it be?"

He reached for his wallet, opened it up and showed me the ten dollars. I was totally puzzled.

"John, what are you looking for?"

"The, the ..." He shaped his hands in a small rectangle. Slowly recognition dawned.

"John, are you looking for these?" I asked as I reached into the glove compartment for the postcards. He hadn't seen me "hide" the postcards, nor had I seen him put the money in his wallet. He nodded as we both laughed at our ridiculous miscommunication and began repacking the car.

While it was a much-needed vacation for both of us, we agreed to set aside two hours every morning to work with the flashcards. At first there were very few he could say alone, and he would have to repeat them after me, if he could. Sometimes even that was too difficult. I soon began to develop short phrases that I would say and he would finish, often from nursery rhymes.

"Jack and Jill went up the ..."

"Hill," he would respond, looking at the flash card.

"Humpty Dumpty sat on the ..."

"Wall," he would say.

"Twinkle, twinkle little ..."

"Star."

I wrote the phrases on post-its attached to the back of each card. Unfortunately, not all the words were easy to match with phrases. Most colors were a challenge as were many of the nouns. I tried many strategies, talking about the word, spelling it, giving him the initial sound, pronouncing the word only as a last resort. After two hours each day, we would stop, whether we had completed all the cards or not. The thing that I found so amazing was that some words were easy some days, other words other days. One day, looking at a card, he would correctly say "orange", the next he might not remember it, and another day he might not even be able to repeat it. I was reminded again that we were going for percentages, rebuilding bridges in his brain. The goal was to be able to increase the number of words that John could say, and the fact that he could say a particular word yesterday was noteworthy, but somewhat irrelevant. I learned later that completing a phrase was a different skill from recognizing and saying the printed word, which was also a different skill from sounding it out, and different again from naming the object, all exercising different areas of the brain. The first was easiest for John, like automatic speech. But I didn't know these things then and I don't know what I would have done differently even if I had known it. I defined success as being able to say a word without my saying it first.

Over the next couple of months as John improved, I made the task more difficult, providing fewer cues, letting him read the phrase on the back of the card silently to fill in the last word. At the end of three months, John was able to say over ninety percent of the words alone, and usually the rest by reading the phrase silently, in a little over an hour.

I have always been a measurement freak. The records I kept for my business were meticulous, not just from an accounting perspective, but also from training and evaluation, marketing and sales, inventory and travel perspectives. It seemed natural to me to keep records of John's improvement. When we first started working with the flashcards, I tracked the method he used to get to each of the correct words. Later, when he could say them, we continued for another month and timed how quickly he could read all 96 cards. Throughout the time we spent working together, I always found myself measuring something. It was second nature to me and made the task more interesting and challenging.

The flashcards were good because I wasn't sure which would help John more, the picture or the word, and I hoped they would reinforce each other. As it turned out, the printed word was what he was saying. The picture helped very little. So we had actually spent most of our effort on sight reading orally. Very little object naming was accomplished.

Once John could say most of the words on the flashcards, I transcribed them into the computer, creating what we called John's dictionary, adding the names of family members, a few verbs and some prepositions, words that he could begin to use to construct sentences. Every day he practiced reading the words aloud. Every few weeks, I wrote down new words and John slowly and laboriously added them to his computer list.

John's object naming was still very poor. Hearing the name of an object and identifying it was difficult. If, for example, I asked him to point to a

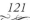

window, he couldn't usually do it. Naming it himself was very rare. He might say, "I'm cold, I need to close it." (meaning the window) The word was not lost, just not accessible when he heard it or wanted to say it. When I wrote down the names of objects in the house on post-its, he would walk around and usually stick them on the correct object—refrigerator, radio, TV, lamp, clock, calendar, window, door. He could understand the word when he read it, but he could not retrieve the word when he wanted to say it. Our house became filled with post-its. But for John to be able to communicate, his speech needed to include self-initiated nouns. Off we went in search of flashcards that only had pictures on the front with the names on the back.

Oral comprehension was an ongoing, every-waking-hour activity. Though John was usually not aware of it, virtually every interaction we had was geared towards improving his oral comprehension. Preparing dinner was a good example. Every night he helped me.

"John, I need an onion. Can you get me an onion?"

"An onion? An onion?" he would repeat, trying to figure out what an onion was.

If that did not produce the desired action, I would continue.

"An onion is a vegetable that you peel and chop up. Sometimes it makes you cry. The onions are in the pantry."

This increased the likelihood that he would find it. If he still couldn't, I would show him where the pantry was. It was possible that by this time, the word pantry had replaced the word onion in his mind and now he did not remember what he was looking for. I would repeat again, "I need an onion." If that failed, I got the onion and showed it to him. We would do this for five or six items every night. Butter, salt and pepper, potatoes, peas, corn, any food we needed. It often seemed as if he was hearing the word for the first time, but, surprisingly, neither of us got frustrated. Of course, it took a little longer to get dinner on the table.

One of John's jobs was to set the table every night, a more difficult assignment than one might imagine. I would tell him and show him if necessary, what we were having for dinner. He would have to figure out what we needed. A fork was a safe bet, but did we need a regular knife or a steak knife? A teaspoon? A soup spoon? Salt and pepper was a safe bet, but what about butter?

We also approached comprehension from a more relaxed, passive perspective. I began reading books to him. John loved mysteries, not my favorite, but a search of the book stores uncovered several books that we thought we could both enjoy. Every month or two, we would select a book that I would read to him in the evenings. John was able to follow the stories and I found myself getting immersed in the plot. He would get tired after about an hour and I forced myself to stop, though I confess to occasionally reading ahead on the sly. This reading time seemed to improve John's comprehension and concentration in a non-threatening way and gave us the opportunity to enjoy a shared experience. Some friends suggested books on tape, but that proved too difficult. When I read to him, he could stop me if he got confused or couldn't remember a character, and we would discuss it. I would explain things in a way he could understand. He couldn't do that with the tapes and after a few attempts with them, he gave up.

In the evenings, we often watched TV. The eleven o'clock news was a regular part of our day. To the extent he was able, John skimmed the newspapers every day, often flagging articles he wanted me to see or to read to him. He began to "read" *People* magazine. It had a lot of pictures and proper nouns and was relatively simple to follow. Sean gave him a subscription for Christmas. I was often amazed by the articles he found and usually willing to read them to him when he asked.

In December, Allison, who was now working with John for two forty-five minute sessions a week, announced that she was leaving to return home to Pennsylvania at the end of the year. A new speech therapist would begin working with John in January. A few weeks into 1998, John decided that he no longer wanted to attend formal sessions.

He was becoming more independent and making more decisions on his own. The independence was crucial to his recovery, but it would lead to the biggest challenge we had faced since his return home.

13

John's Driving Need

By January, 1998, John wanted to drive. The more he recovered, the more important his independence became. Where we lived, driving was essential for functional independence. His license would expire that October and I knew he would be required, at a minimum, to undergo an eye test. It was important to renew it before it expired because I didn't know if he would ever be able to take a written exam.

In August of 1997, four months after the stroke, an eye examination by Dr. Kelman, a neuro-ophthalmologist affiliated with the University of Maryland Medical System, indicated that John's vision was improving. He was regaining sight in the upper right quadrant of both eyes and could expect continued improvement for at least the first year. The doctor had been optimistic and over time, I could tell John's vision was getting better. I wasn't sure if his eyes were good enough to pass the eye exam, but I knew his speech wasn't.

The standard eye test consisted of reading the letters on a chart, something that John couldn't do. Reciting the entire alphabet was automatic, being able to point to one letter and say it was not. So we established as one of our objectives being able to name the letters of the alphabet. We had nine months to work on it before his license would expire.

In late January, we took a three week trip to Florida, needing the warmth and sun and freedom of the outdoors that Florida offered that time of year. It was in Florida that we began the task of learning the alphabet, the most difficult and discouraging of the jobs we attempted. Maybe I went about it completely wrong, feeling for the first time the added pressure of having a deadline. Certainly I underestimated how difficult it would be.

We started with the letter "M". It was a frequently used letter and seemed as good a place to start as any. We would add one new letter every day, until he could recognize the entire alphabet. I wrote the letter "M" on an index card. I would say "em", he would repeat it. We were driving around the state and there were plenty of opportunities to see the letter in print—Motel, Mobil, Movie... He taped the card to the dashboard where he could see it. He searched for Mobil stations. About every ten minutes, I asked him what the letter was. He couldn't remember. I repeated "em". He repeated it. Sometimes when he found a Mobil station, he could say "Mobil". If I immediately asked him what the letter was, he could make the sound "mmm", the starting sound of the word Mobil, but not name the letter. At least a hundred times that first day, I asked him what the letter was. He correctly identified it less than five times. Enough for the first day. Maybe he'd remember it better if he slept on it.

The next day, we started again with "M". Day Two was no better. At the end of the day, he was still unable to look at the index card and say "M". To say I was discouraged and frustrated would be a gross understatement. I felt myself getting angry and irritable, not the best mood for a vacation. Maybe we had started with a letter that was too hard. Are some letters harder than others? Maybe he needed to start with a letter in which the sound it made was the same as the initial sound of its name, like "T". Now we had two letters taped to the dashboard. We began our search of Texaco stations as well as Mobil stations. We never had to wait long to find one. Knowing how John related to numbers, I made the mistake of singing "Tea for two, and two for tea" a few times. For the rest of the day, the letter "T" was pronounced "two". By nightfall I was at the end of my rope.

The third day ended with us no closer to getting a single letter learned. At least when I said the letter "M" or "T", he could usually point to the correct one, but he couldn't say it. It must be my fault. What was I doing wrong? What should I do differently? That night I wrote out the pronunciation of all the letters and discovered a few basic categories and some exceptions. Maybe I should forget letters like "M" that were pronounced by starting with a short vowel sound and instead concentrate on letters whose initial sound was the sound made by the letter and that ended with a long e sound. So I had T, B, D, G, P, V and Z to work with. Day Four we tried "T" and "P", over and over. John got discouraged but I tried to be positive, assuring him that he would get it, that it was just taking a little longer than we expected.

Secretly I was afraid that we had attempted something that was too difficult for John, but I didn't have the heart to tell him that he might not be able to learn the alphabet. He was trying so hard. The task had become equally trying, but I pretended everything was fine. We seemed to have come up against a brick wall. Ten months had elapsed since his stroke. Several of the doctors had said that we could expect recovery to continue for a year after his stroke. Had he recovered all he could? Was this what he was left with? How would he feel about that?

We had believed that if we just kept working at it, he would keep getting better. Unable to sleep that night, I wondered if we were wrong. How many more times could I point to the letter "T" and ask him what it was, and have him not be able to say it, or say "two" without screaming at him? Patience was still a goal, not a virtue of mine. My rose-colored glasses were clouding up. I had believed earlier that if John never got any better than he was at Kernan, it would be all right. Now I was being put to the test. Could I really accept it? Just four months earlier, I had closed my office, expecting to dedicate my time to John's recovery, "our new job", I thought with gallows humor. Please God, don't let it be over so soon. I was close to despair.

There was no question that John was a wonderful person. There was no question that I loved him and was loved in return. He wanted so much to learn, but was it kind or cruel to keep pushing him? Was I selfish to not be satisfied? Was I doing something wrong? I cursed his "broken bridges". That night in the hotel, laying in the dark beside my sleeping husband, it seemed so unfair. Not the stroke. I had accepted that, though that too was certainly unfair. It was the brick wall. John was not failing here, I was, and it was my failure that depressed me. I believed that he would keep getting better. Now I wasn't sure. How many times do you hit your head against a brick wall before you give up? Should we quit? Could we quit? Was John as frustrated as I was? I couldn't ask him, afraid of his answer. I was frustrated and depressed and felt guilty.

It wasn't the alphabet. By itself, the alphabet was irrelevant. It was the eye exam for the driving test. If John couldn't pass the eye exam, I didn't think they'd let him drive and if he couldn't identify the letters, I didn't think he would pass the eye exam. Driving was so important to him. It brought with it such tremendous freedom. I couldn't bear to see him fail. Mary, mother of God, what should I do?

Morning finally dawned. I suggested to John that we take the day off, enjoy the vacation, not worry about the alphabet for a day. I couldn't tell him that I couldn't deal with it just yet. That day, we walked along the beach, browsed through the shops, dined out and never mentioned the alphabet once.

I didn't have the guts to tell him that it seemed too difficult for him, that maybe we should stop. Perhaps cowardice, in its way, is a virtue. Perhaps Mary was looking over my shoulder when the next day, reluctantly and with a great deal of dread, I pointed to the letter "T" on the dashboard as we began driving.

"Do you know what letter this is?"

"T," he responded.

"Do you know what letter this is?" I asked, pointing to the letter "P".

"P?" he asked.

Was this a fluke? Would he forget them in a few minutes or did he know them? I tried "M". He made the sound "mmm". Forget "M". I pulled off the road, grabbed an index card and wrote "B". He recognized it as the second letter of the alphabet and could repeat it consistently. I wondered if there were other letters he just knew. Pulling into a parking lot, I wrote each letter on an index card, mixed them up and asked him to name any letters he could. He named several—A, B, C, P, T, V, W, X, and Z. He recognized the letters near the front and end of the alphabet. I had been trying to teach him letters in the middle—apparently the hardest for him. I felt stupid because I knew that a good teacher builds on what the learner already knows. How could I have forgotten it? Why had I not checked to see which ones he already knew?

With renewed enthusiasm and determination, we started again. I collected the cards with the letters he already knew. That was our starting point. Each day, after reviewing the letters he knew, we added letters from the beginning and end of the alphabet as he seemed ready, gradually working towards the middle which was more difficult. We had gotten around the brick wall. By mid-April, John could correctly say all the letters in the alphabet with about ninety percent accuracy.

In late April, he met with the neuro-ophthalmologist again to have his eyes reexamined. One year had elapsed since his stroke. Not only had his vision improved significantly, but he correctly identified every letter on the eye chart. The previous August, the doctor had been unable to test his vision, since John couldn't name any letters, couldn't tell the doctor what he saw, couldn't follow his commands and only seemed able to indicate that either things kept disappearing or he saw two or four of them. And his speech was jargon. Now he could read the eye chart correctly, take the field of view test, and answer his questions. Dr. Kelman was astonished. He wrote in his report:

"Since the last visit, the patient has had remarkable recovery. He is now able to recognize all the letters. His speech is clearly more fluent. He is now able to perform the Snellen visual acuity testing and his vision is normal. He has definitely made improvements."

His field of view had improved as well. The doctor gave us a certificate that we could present to the Motor Vehicle Administration in lieu of his taking their eye test.

John's experience with the alphabet taught me three things, all of which I thought I already knew. The first is that learning never stops. It may plateau. It may look like it stopped. Be patient. It will resume. This lesson I will never again doubt.

The second is that when you encounter a brick wall and find yourself hitting your head against it, stop. Stand back and see if you can go around it or over it. Brick walls are hard to smash through. The goal is to get to the other side not to make a hole in the wall. More than once, in my single-minded focus, I lost sight of the goal. Rather than insisting he learn the letters I selected, I should have built upon what he already knew. I kept

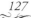
trying to figure out how to smash through the wall. Perhaps I was the one with a vision problem!

The third falls loosely in the category of miracles. I'm not concerned with the church's definition here. I'm talking about your everyday miracles—the miracle of a new idea that seems to solve the unsolvable problem, the miracle of not being able to give up when you don't see progress, the miracle of hope. Trust in miracles.

Armed with the eye certificate, I was still nervous. The law in Maryland requires that, following a stroke, the patient must notify the Division of Motor Vehicles (DMV) and a doctor must certify in writing that the patient has recovered sufficiently to drive. Rather than ignore the law and discover sometime in the future that his automobile insurance would be invalid if he was involved in an accident, I spoke with Dr. LaMonte. Her letter stopped short of certifying him, stating only that he had a stoke and had passed an eye examination for driving.

To cover my bases, I went alone to a DMV field office where drivers licenses were renewed and asked a woman there if there would be any problems for "a friend" who had a stoke and needed to renew his license. She asked if he was physically disabled. I told her he wasn't and volunteered that he had passed the required eye exam, but had residual communication difficulties, particularly with his speech. She said speech wasn't a criteria for driving and she didn't see why there should be a problem.

As soon as John received his notice to renew, we went to the local DMV office and waited nervously in line. He finally stepped up to the teller, handed her his renewal form, the certification which would bypass their eye exam, and the doctor's letter. The woman behind the counter read the brief letter, handed it to a teller beside her and asked what she was supposed to do with it. The second woman shrugged and said it should probably be sent to the main office. I was afraid that would delay everything, but she proceeded to process his application, then sent him to the cashier to accept payment, before getting his picture taken. All the months of work and worry evaporated as John sat, waiting for his new license to be issued. Sending the letter to DMV headquarters should bury it forever, I thought as I realized she had never seen such a letter before. Apparently few people knew or followed the law, but we had chosen to play it safe. John was a legal driver! We went out to celebrate.

Two months later, John received a letter from the DMV requiring that he submit to a brake reaction test and a driving test or his license would be suspended. So much for burying paperwork! Other than explaining to him what was involved in the brake reaction test in which John would see a green light while his foot rested on a simulated gas pedal on the floor, and would then have to "brake" when the light turned red, there was nothing we could do to prepare for it. To prepare for the driving test, we drove around the neighborhood, while I told him where to turn. With no cars around, he frequently failed to use his turn signals, insisting there was no one to see them. So we had the "turn-signal fight". He practiced parallel parking with his tiny Miata after I procured orange cones to mark off the space. Though parallel parking is rarely required in the suburbs where we live, John was a native New Yorker and could have done it blindfolded. He did argue that I put the cones too close together, and so we had the "cone-placement" fight. John was definitely getting more feisty! Those fights, though heated, were short in duration and always ended with laughter over the silliness of them, and assurances of continued love.

John passed the brake reaction test with near perfect times, well above the requirement of the test, but did lose 2 points for failure to use his blinker signal once. He was now fully approved by DMV to drive, a certified legal driver, and though his driving was generally restricted to local stores and occasional weekday masses, John had achieved the independence he needed, deserved, and had worked so hard to achieve. We had both succeeded.

14

Life After Stroke—The Search for Independence

Sometimes John drove me absolutely crazy. Were I to be fair at this point, I would have to concede that it's possible that I might have driven him crazy too—and it was usually about the same thing. Perseveration of thought—where the brain gets an idea locked in and can't seem to let it go. In a normal person, I'd probably call it obsessing, although one might argue that being obsessive negates normalcy. Anyway, John would get an idea locked in his head and couldn't let it go until it was resolved. He'd decide he wanted to get the oil changed in his car, or he wanted to buy stamps, or milk, or he wanted me to call someone on the phone, or any one of a hundred things.

My track record on automobile maintenance is far from sterling, and to me, changing the oil is an unnecessary inconvenience. John is an every-three-thousand-miles-oil-changing fanatic. When I would agreed to do it, I meant I'd think about getting around to it sometime soon. John meant call right now and make an appointment. He'd bug me until I did it, so the appointment was often made under duress just to get him off my back. Sometimes it was easier to go to the grocery store twice a day, once for milk and later for bananas, than to listen to the same requests over and over. Making lists of John's requests seemed to help but then I still had to do the things on the list, regardless of how unimportant they were to me, because John could not get them out of his mind until they were resolved. Eventually, John began to make grocery lists by copying the name of items from their packaging. It wasn't always the right words and made for some odd lists. "Kodak" meant film, "dry roasted" meant peanuts, "2%" meant milk and "extra virgin" (I hope!) meant olive oil.

But I had my insidious ways of getting revenge. John's most frequent driving complaint was my failure to downshift when the car slowed. He would look frustrated or disgusted and point to the stick shift, occasionally saying, "Pop it." I told him if he was going to complain about my driving, he had to use correct English; he had to say, "change gears", or I would ignore him. Suffice it to say he eventually learned to say "change gears", although the process was painful for both of us.

Writing checks was a monthly activity that I always dreaded. It wasn't the money. I just hated taking the time to do it. So we began to set aside one morning a month to write checks. I would balance the checkbook and go through the bills that had to be paid. I had converted most of the monthly bills to automatic deductions from our checking account, the mortgage, the utilities, the phone bill. John would write the checks for the newspapers, the credit cards, magazine renewals, charities and other miscellaneous payments. He would copy the name of the organization and the amount to be paid from the bill, and then use a chart to lookup the amount in words, (i.e. two hundred fifty three) to complete the second line on the check. He would copy the account number on the bottom left corner, sign it and prepare the envelope. I checked everything before it was mailed. Writing these few checks took a couple of hours, but it seemed like a necessary step towards independence.

John didn't remember any of his old pin numbers. We went to our bank and selected one that would be easy for him to remember so he could use his ATM card at the bank, the grocery store and for other shopping. We tried to use it at least a couple of times a month, but it was too difficult. Each machine required slightly different input. Even inserting the card correctly so the magnetic strip could be read was a challenge. If he was too slow some machines recycled and he had to start again, which really confused him. When the bank, and later our grocery store updated their machines and changed the questions and order of responses, I almost went ballistic. Why can't they standardize? It is a continual reminder to me of how difficult and unforgiving the electronic world has become to people who are challenged as John is. So I still needed to be with him when he used it, and bank trips or grocery shopping were still joint ventures when he didn't have enough cash.

John found a good way to handle grocery lists. He would scan the weekly grocery flyer circling items he wanted to buy. I would circle others, perhaps adding a few items at the top of the front page. Flyer in hand, he would go alone and search the shelves for the items he wanted, crossing them off as he added them to his cart. Usually he found most of them, only occasionally the wrong brand, and would show the flyer to an employee when he needed help. It was a clever solution to his problem of not being able to either say the word or match the written word to the item he wanted. It brought him more independence and a great deal of pride in each weekly success.

Once John began making his own trips to the grocery store and post office, the gas station and hardware store, the people he dealt with were marvelous. Our postmasters Carol and Bill are good examples. The post office in our little town of Highland is probably unique in this age of automation and impersonalization. Carol and Bill seem to know everyone and greet them by name. They decorate their tiny space for the holidays and put out treats for special days like Valentine's Day, tax day, and Halloween. Just before Easter, a six foot bunny will be dispensing stamps with candy and Santa Claus makes his appearance behind the counter before Christmas. They make going to the post office a pleasurable experience. Carol knew that John had a stroke. One day when John and I stopped in together, the three of us discussed what was easy and what was hard for him. Once he was driving again, he would go into the post office to mail a package, buy stamps, request that they hold the mail or pick it up after a trip. Occasionally I would write a note. If he needed help, they helped him, always patient and understanding, never condescending. They treated him as a pleasant, cheerful customer and neighbor. Driving gave John independence. Wonderful people helped him to exercise it.

John greeted everyone with a cheerful "Good morning." This was fine as long as it was before noon. He did get strange looks from clerks in the afternoon and waiters at dinner, but no amount of correcting seemed to help. It was an automatic greeting and he could not switch to "good afternoon" or "hello" easily. It would bother me if someone laughed, but somehow it wasn't worth explaining to every stranger that he'd had a stroke. I would correct him privately but the odd impression had already been made. Sometimes I would remind him as we approached someone to say hello rather than good morning, but occasionally he still slipped. It wasn't often, and over time it didn't matter so much anymore.

Dr. Marian LaMonte put us in touch with Dr. Steve Small, a professor in the Department of Neurology at the University of Maryland Medical System who was doing research in the area of cognitive neuroscience and neurorehabilitation because she thought that John might be a good subject for his research. We were excited about the possibility of participating in their research, studying physical recovery from stroke, but after a few meetings and tests, they decided that John was not a good candidate for their project and for months we heard no more. But as a result of that encounter, in the spring of 1998, Dr. Small referred us to Dr. Rita Berndt in the same department to see if John might be a good candidate for a language research project they were conducting. Charlotte Mitchum, a speech language pathologist involved in the language research project contacted us and we began to meet weekly with her in her office in downtown Baltimore. For months, she tested every aspect of John's communication skills and identified specific areas of learning which she and John would focus on.

Because John showed a remarkable pattern of recovery, Dr. Small and Dr. Martha Burton continued to follow his progress with neuro-imaging techniques that were just evolving at the time. They wanted to monitor John to see if they could correlate changes in his language over time to changes in brain activity. John agreed to participate and spent many hours in the MRI as they conducted tests before, during and after specific learning objectives were met with Charlotte. The possibility that we might be able to physically see changes in John's brain as he relearned language skills was fascinating to us, and John was pleased to be able to make some contribution to the eventual understanding of how stroke-induced brain damage can alter one's ability to think and communicate.

I attended John's weekly meeting with Charlotte because none of us felt comfortable with him driving alone into Baltimore. We liked Charlotte immensely and both looked forward to the sessions. She made it clear from the beginning that the purpose of these sessions was research, not therapy and that John might personally get little benefit from the study. John had already stopped his formal speech therapy sessions and we were working alone at home. We both believed that John would benefit from his time with her and we were truly interested in the prospect of contributing to a better understanding of the problems caused by aphasia. While John and I focused on reading at home, much of her emphasis was on comprehension and speech. Even after a year of living with John's stroke, I was often amazed by things that she discovered were easy for him, and things that were difficult. She helped us understand which problems were common for stroke survivors and which ones were unique to John. She pointed out that John was fortunate because he had the ability to relearn and adapt. This made him a good candidate for language therapy research. She had worked with other stroke survivors, some as motivated as John, who did not have this ability. While I was often frustrated by how long it took for John to learn something, she was amazed that he could relearn. It helped to put things in perspective. Charlotte often suggested ways I could work with John at home when I wasn't sure I was doing the right thing. While we were careful to avoid the areas she focused on during their sessions together, we implemented her ideas in reading. She even provided us with good reading material.

John's sessions with Charlotte were usually Wednesday mornings from ten to noon. Our treat after that was to dine at *Donna's*, a restaurant in the hospital where the portobello mushroom and goat cheese salad became our standing order. These weekly outings were both beneficial and fun. After the first year, John began driving himself to these sessions and had lunch alone at *Donna's* where they considered him a regular. John loved the freedom and independence associated with going alone and eating out. As with each step toward independence, we followed a process. In the case of driving to Baltimore, first I drove him many times. Then, for several trips, I sat in the passenger seat as he drove. On his first trip alone, I called Charlotte before he left. She called me when he arrived. After that we agreed to work by exception processing. We would only call if John wasn't on time.

As John began to relearn specific tasks, MRIs showed new areas of activity on the right side of his brain, that mirrored where activity would have been expected on the left side, had his brain not been damaged. Even at his age, the right side was taking up some of the workload.

After John's stroke, we considered moving to a warmer climate. Neither of us liked cold weather, so one of the reasons for our trips to the southwest and to Florida had been to check them out. We decided to stay where we were. We liked our house. We had friends and some family here. John's mom was only four hours away. So, in the spring of 1998, we began a series of renovations to make the house more compatible with our new life style. In the family room where we spent most of our time, we converted our leaky wood fireplace into an efficient gas fireplace. We added a gas fireplace in our bedroom and in the sunroom, so those rooms would be warmer without having to heat unused space. We remodeled our bathroom and bedroom. Though John had recovered physically from his stroke, with each change, we wanted to include improvements that would make our house more accessible to someone with physical limitations and more comfortable for us. The shower was enlarged and a bench seat and a handheld spray were added. Where feasible, doors were widened, carpet replaced with hardwood.

We both participated in the planning and decorating, but most of the work was contracted. Since we needed living space while the work was in progress, we decided to implement the improvements in a series of steps. The downside was that the work took several months to complete. Our garage took on the appearance of a junk yard—some items waiting to be trashed, some donated to charity, some supplies waiting to be used in the next phase of the renovation, some left over from the last phase that I, being a pack rat, could not bear to throw away. During this time, John's car was parked in the driveway, and maneuvering around the renovation materials in the garage presented an unnecessary challenge to him. John asked me many times to throw it all out. I told him to be patient. Finally he exploded.

Sixteen months had elapsed since John's stroke. Not once had he raised his voice to me in anger. Not much seemed to upset him. Suddenly he began using words that had been long absent from his vocabulary. He was furious. He wanted this junk gone! He wanted to put his car in the garage. Four letter words emerged. New nouns and adjectives emerged. At first I was shocked, then astonished at his temper. Then at his vocabulary. He was frustrated by my apparent indifference to the mess in the garage. Instinctively I was defensive, then angry, then guilty. He was right. There was a lot we could do to clean up the garage but it just hadn't been important enough to me. I stormed into the house. John continued his ranting in the garage.

As I listened to his angry words, I was struck by how clearly he was speaking. I began to laugh. He continued, unaware of my laughter. He must be getting better. This must be part of getting better. Lord help me, he's getting better. I left him alone, afraid to let him see me laughing. It took him nearly twenty minutes to calm down. Well, he was right and I still loved him. I went out to tell him that. He said he still loved me too. Neither of us stayed angry. Had this scene occurred before his stroke, regardless of what he said, I would have heard that he hated me and for at least a week, we wouldn't have spoken to each other or shared a bed. Now I heard that he hated the mess in the garage. It amazed me how much better we could fight when we knew we loved each other. That week we worked together to clean out the garage and John moved his car back into it. Fighting, although we don't do it often, had become a safer thing to do. We could both get mad, say rotten things and apologize. It was okay to fight. Love sure changed the equation. So does saying you're sorry, or admitting the other person is right. Why was it so hard before?

As John's reading progressed, his dictionary grew to over 700 words and we began to read only a part of it every day. At Charlotte's suggestion, we moved on to children's books. We started with simple books having only a few words on each page, then moved up to more challenging ones. We selected common childhood stories like Cinderella and Pinocchio, fairy tales and stories that John remembered. I usually timed these activities, counting the number of words he read and the amount of time it took to read them. After collecting the data for months, not having any idea what I would do with it, I entered it on a spreadsheet and found that the common element was words per hour and it could be plotted on a graph. Instinctively I knew that some days were better than others, but plotting it provided remarkable data. The graph began in January 1998, nine months after his stroke, when John read 71 words per hour from the flashcards. Within a few months, using the reading list, the rate had tripled to about 200 words per hour on average. By the end of 1998, he was reading from the list at over 500 words per hour, occasionally reaching up to 600. With the children's stories I found much greater variability. Some stories were harder than others, but by late spring, reading books at about second grade level, John was averaging over 1500 words per hour. By my measurements, John's reading had improved twenty-fold in sixteen months and was continuing to improve two years after his stroke.

Although, reading out loud, John's speed increased from 71 words per hour to 1500 in less than a year and a half, it was still a slow, halting process. For comparison, when I read one of his stories at a normal "story-telling" speed, it was almost seven times faster, over 10,000 words per hour. There was still a long way to go. There were some words he almost always knew, some he never seemed to learn, but it was more often a random process, recognizing them one time and then not knowing them when they appeared only a few words later. As before, the goals were to increase the probability of recognizing and saying the word, and to increase his consistency.

As his reading improved, I timed him less frequently. It made reading more fun when we also talked about the story. And as the stories got longer, I got tired of counting the number of words every day.

The data was never intended to be used for scientific analysis, so some days I helped him more than others. The controls placed on this measurement process were not rigid, but I believe that the general conclusions are valid. John's reading skills continued to improve measurably. Contrary to what many doctors have concluded, recovery doesn't have to stop after some period of time. Bad days may follow good days for no apparent reason and it can be discouraging. Our experience has proven that good days will come and they excite and encourage us. We also discovered that if we stopped for a few weeks, John regressed and we had to work hard for at least a week to bring his reading back up again.

John's reading chart looked a lot like the graph of the Dow Jones Industrial Average during the 90's. Some days, the DJIA changed by 10 points, more often by 50. It was not unusual to see a change of over 100 points, occasionally more. Every single day it changed—either up or down. So did John's reading speed. But John and I were not day traders in either the stock market or the recovery process. John's recovery, like our portfolio, is a lifetime investment. We knew that our strategy would pay off over time, and require a lot of patience. As long as we believed that the strategy was sound, even when the short-term return was less than we hoped for, the program continued. We never knew how the next day would be. But the trend was definitely good and the effort was unquestionably worth it.

Traveling became an important part of our life. In June 1998 we spent three weeks in Ireland and visited John's cousin there. Sean graduated from University of New Mexico in December, so Albuquerque was back on the itinerary. January of 1999 was spent in Hawaii, May was spent visiting John's boys out west and his brother in Dubuque. In September, John and I went to California to see my sons who were now living together in San Jose. These trips were punctuated with shorter visits to John's family in New York and my parents in Florida. Everywhere we went, we planned the trips together, deciding which route to take, which nights to splurge, which nights to conserve our financial resources. We almost always agreed and we always had fun. "Trip fights", common before his stroke, were few and far between. The new trip fight, which we had at many an airport in the country, was triggered by his decision to go to the men's room seconds before the gate attendant began boarding. The fact that we'd been sitting at the gate for forty five minutes waiting to board didn't seem to matter. I didn't want to give him his boarding pass and board without him, hoping he'd find his way back. I didn't want to be the last person to board, unable to find an overhead compartment for our luggage. After a couple of panic attacks on my part when John wandered off and took a long time to return, I got very angry. Faced with the options I offered him, divorce, castration, or going to the rest room ten minutes before scheduled boarding time, he opted for the last one. Still, whenever they announced our row to board, he would tell me he needed to go to the bathroom, and grin—just to bug me. It worked.

John's mother died February 1999. It was sudden and we weren't there. Fortunately, John and I had just visited her a couple of weeks earlier. She was a good, kind and loving woman, and is very much missed. She had been so supportive of John's recovery, and had written to him weekly after his stroke. She could barely see to write and John could barely read. What a loving pair they made. On the last evening of her wake, after friends had left and only family remained in the room, John stood before the gathering and read a short prepared statement I had helped him compose and rehearse.

"Mom, I love you. When I was a kid, you were always there for me. As a father, and after my stroke, you were there to help me. I know you are happy with pop now, but you will always be with me too."

He was distraught, and beyond the first sentence many of the words were transposed. When he finished the room was silent, tears streaming down everyone's faces. I went up to hug him. Still no one moved. Brendan walked up. "Good man," he said as he hugged him. Everyone still sat, suspended in time, paralyzed. His daughter Janet walked over and hugged him tightly. John, sensing the tension in the air, looked as if life was being squeezed out of him, grinned, and in a plaintive cry directed at Janet's tight hold on him, said to the crowd, "Help me, help me." Janet let go. Everyone in the room burst into laughter. The tension was gone and we could all breathe again. John's humor had rescued us. He has a way of doing that.

The Spring 1999 catalog from our local community college arrived in late February. I always enjoyed looking through the catalog. Both John and I had taken a few courses over the years. John took courses in foreign languages and travel, while I opted for classes like financial investing and home remodeling. We had never attended together and usually we were either too busy or traveling too frequently to sign up for anything. Now we had time. Maybe we could take one together. I made a mental list of all the criteria this course would have to satisfy. It couldn't require a lot of reading. There could be no written assignments, no oral presentations. There could be no writing in class, like taking notes. Class discussion should not be required. The class should be relaxing and non-threatening. A small class would be best. Other than auto repair, which didn't interest either of us, and aerobics, which wasn't my idea of fun, there wasn't much left. My criteria had ruled out just about everything—until I found what I thought was perfect—a massage class. I always wanted to be married to a man who could give a good massage! John, though less enthusiastic, agreed. There were only four sessions, no reading, no homework, no class discussion—perfect.

We brought our supplies to the first class—pillows, massage oil, towels. The class had twelve students. After we listened to a short lecture, we watched the demonstration. Now we would take turns massaging each other, focusing on the legs and feet. I massaged John as the instructor therapist verbally directed us. No problem, John loved it. We reversed roles.

The therapist began again, "Form a V with your palm and index finger. With your palm down, rub along the shin bone from the ankle to the knee."

John's face puzzled over. What's a "V" look like? He had to think. What's a palm? Fingers are those things on your hand, right? But what's an index finger? What's a shin? Where's the ankle? The knee? The instruction was impossible for John to comprehend, much less to follow. There were too many words, each of which his brain had to contemplate, to repeat and organize into a coherent whole.

How could I have spent so much effort looking for the perfect class and yet forgotten that he didn't know body parts? John was totally perplexed and tried to imitate the other students, but positioned at the end of the row, his back now to the group, it was difficult for him to observe them without completely turning around. They, of course, were all facing us, watching the bizarre charades.

Even the words he recognized were switched in his head. Knee and elbow, at the moment, were interchanged. So while his mind was telling him to do one thing, the other students were doing something else. While he rubbed his hand from my shoulder to my elbow, everyone else was massaging legs. Trying not to embarrass him or arouse the attention of the other students, I tried to point him in the direction of my leg with the arm he now held captive, whispering loudly to move lower, realizing he didn't know what lower meant, using my head and eyes to gesture that it was down *there*, not up *here*. Even if he didn't know what an index finger and a palm were, if he would just do something to my leg instead of my arm, maybe we wouldn't look so strange. After what seemed like hours, but was probably less than two minutes, I began to feel like I was part of an "I Love Lucy" comedy show. Lucy had those saucer eyes that conveyed guilt and cover up each time she found herself in over her head, knowing she'd screwed up, pretending everything was fine, as she frantically tried to fake it. At break I knew I needed to speak with the instructor. She had been watching our massage folly curiously. I was surprised and relieved to learn that she was also a nurse who had worked for years with stroke patients. She understood the problem and by the next class had a solution.

Thereafter, whenever it was John's turn to massage me, she would come over and do to my left arm or leg, whatever John was supposed to do to my right, while she instructed the class. John could watch her easily and imitate her movements. And I got a double massage. Great solution, but I sure felt foolish! To my mental list of criteria for future classes, I added, "Can't require knowledge of body parts."

Decision making was another area that was difficult for John. In May of 1999 when we were in Las Vegas visiting John Andrew, our hotel had a spectacular breakfast buffet. Usually when we dine out, John orders one of three things, fresh tuna, chicken or whatever I'm having. I attribute that to the fact that he doesn't know what the other items are, whether he reads them or I read them to him, so he orders something safe. If he saw the foods, he could have fun exploring his options. This buffet offered a forty-foot-long array of choices. Given the assortment of juices, fruits, breads, yogurt, oatmeal, muesli, and toppings, John kept returning to the buffet unable to decide what he wanted, each time selecting a small amount of one or two dishes. And that was before he got to the main course items. People make life-altering decisions faster than John selected his breakfast items. John enjoyed it, but if we were going to do this again, I'd allow a lot more time and pace my own eating better. I probably gained five pounds as I nibbled away the hour and a half it took John to create a modest breakfast.

As a result of his stroke, John's personality changed. Not completely of course, but he is different. I can't explain or even understand many of the changes that took place in John's brain. But I can observe them and describe them, not as a doctor or a researcher, but as a wife, as someone who was close to him and saw the changes. There are so many traits that we attribute, both correctly and incorrectly to men or to women. We may say "men are more analytical" or "women tend to be more intuitive". At the same time, we recognize that there are so many exceptions that it may seem to invalidate the rule we put forth. Society attributes these characteristics to both heredity and environment. Chemicals and hormones seem to explain some behavioral changes. Pictures of the brain overlay functions with specific locations in the brain—speech in one place, feeling in another. We talk about left-brain and right-brain activities and generalize that men are more left-brained, women are more right-brained. Newer research seems to point to a highly complex network of activity going on, crossing boundaries between the left and right side of the brain. What I do know is that John suffered massive damage to the left side of his brain. After his stroke and initial recovery, there were still severe cognitive and communication deficits. But his personality changed too. Had he become more "right-brained"? Maybe. Were there chemical changes that occurred as a result of his stroke? Maybe. Were there a hundred other things that could account for the changes? Maybe.

But he is different and I like the difference. He is nicer, happier, less aggressive, less critical. He is more affectionate, more demonstrative, more appreciative, more sensitive. He is quicker to praise, slower to anger. He is more willing to join in whatever activity I suggest. He is unquestionably easier to love.

In many ways, however, he did not change. His sense of humor is completely intact. So is his memory for everything except language. He is still responsible and dependable and if he promises to do something, he'd do it. He still loves to travel, still enjoys the outdoors, still wants to get physical exercise every day. He seems happy to be alive and his joy is contagious.

His speech has improved but many distinctions are lost on him. For example, he interchanges words ending in "ed" and "ing". My favorite misspeak occurs when something amazes him and he exclaims, "I'm amazing."

"Yes, John," I can honestly reply with a grin, "that is true."

Several friends and relatives have asked if they could trade places with me, or at least borrow my husband for a while. They wish they had husbands who held their hand, who told them every day how much they loved them, who bragged about their wives to anyone who would listen. People tell me how lucky I am. They're right.

In September 1999, John saw a picture in a magazine of a car that he said was really neat. The new Chrysler PT Cruiser was designed to look like a car from the 1930's. John said it reminded him of his father. Years ago, John bought a Cadillac for his father, who loved the car, drove it proudly and kept it in pristine condition. John derived pleasure from witnessing his father's. John mentioned that he might like to buy this new Chrysler.

John keeps cars for a long time. He'd been driving his Miata convertible for ten years and it looked brand new. The Chrysler was probably safer than the Miata. He would soon receive money from his parent's estate, and if the car reminded him of his parents, that might be a good use for some of the money. A few evenings after that discussion we drove to a Chrysler dealer to see if they had one, not realizing it wouldn't be available for months. The dealer was closed and we didn't see any in the window, but I promised we would come back. A project for another time.

A few days passed. John ran an errand to purchase some supplies for the fish pond. He was gone a long time and I began to worry, but John would often make side trips to the grocer or gas station. I was in the basement when he finally arrived.

"John, are you all right? I was beginning to worry."

"Well, sort of."

"Sort of? Did you get hurt?"

"No, I'm fine."

"Did you have a problem with the car?"

"Not exactly."

"Not exactly? John, what happened?"

"I bought a car."

"No, John, you didn't buy a car. Do you mean you bought *gas* for the car?" John often misspoke and this would be typical of such a statement.

"No, I bought a car."

"No, John, you don't mean you bought a *car*. You mean you bought *gas* for the car."

"No, I bought a car," he insisted and handed me the sales receipt.

I was dumbfounded. Then I started to laugh. "You bought a car? You bought a car without me? You really bought a car?" I couldn't stop laughing. I couldn't believe it. He had walked into the dealer, somehow described the car, seen pictures of it, discovered it wouldn't be available until Spring of 2000, found out the approximate price, selected the color and gave them a deposit with his VISA. John bought a car. All by himself. Without me. I was astonished, amazed, delighted, amused, and shocked. Our goal had been independence. I wasn't sure I was ready for it.

15

Success is a Journey

As I close this book, three years have elapsed since that awful day in April 1997. What is John like now? Physically, his health is excellent, with no hint of the paralysis that temporarily imprisoned him. The sparkle in his eyes has returned and his face has all the animation it ever possessed. Short of a yet undiscovered medical miracle, we will live with the aphasia that impairs his communication skills forever. He can read aloud, haltingly, at about a third grade level. We believe this will continue to improve with hard work. His speech is devoid of many verbs, and most nouns, but words he has not uttered since his stroke continue to emerge. John's casual, automatic speech is fluent and most people initially detect no problem. Charlotte once said that someone engaging him in conversation for the first time might assume he had a stutter rather than realizing the magnitude of his loss. He often says the opposite of what he means—a puzzling though apparently common phenomenon that I have come to accept, but one that can be confusing and frustrating for both of us in daily living. Little effort has been spent on learning to write again, so little progress has been made. A job for the future perhaps. John's comprehension of what he hears is good for simple things, but he can be easily confused as complexity increases or if he feels rushed. And filtering is still a problem. If several people are talking, John can't separate one voice from the others and listen to it.

The hot-cold thing hasn't worked out so well. Before John's stroke, I was always cold, he was hot. The thermostat was a common battle scene. Afterwards, we were cold together. I thought it was great. But I discovered as I go through menopause, that now I'm hot and he's cold. It would have been more convenient temperature-wise if he could have waited to have his stroke until my hot flashes were over. Now I kick off the covers that John is burrowed under and we're fighting over the thermostat again.

Because my background was in software development, I liken the way his brain processes data to a software program. Ten to twenty percent of the software that is written is needed to handle normal, routine processing—when everything works the way it's supposed to, as it does most of the time. The other eighty to ninety percent of code is created to deal with the exceptions, unexpected or rare events (like Y2K), erroneous data, human error—the things we never thought of or never thought would happen, the ones we're not prepared for. This code in software is often untested, faulty, or missing. Processing of exceptions is usually the weakest part of a program. So it is with John. His normal, everyday processing works fairly well. Exception processing, like when the pharmacy can't fill the prescription, or a bill is incorrect, or the debit machine is different in every store—those things are too difficult. A simple everyday example is that he can point to a salad on the menu, and sometimes say it, but not ask for salad dressing on the side.

How does John perceive all this? I asked him again to tell me what he remembers of the early days after his stroke. Each time he is able to tell me more, not because he remembers more, but because his ability to describe it improves. Because his speech often rambles, I have excerpted parts of his story and summarized others. Direct quotes are from a tape he made recently. Words in italics are exactly his, those in parentheses are my descriptions of his gestures or the word I think he means.

John describes the night he had the stroke.

"Well, I knew exactly what, where.. and I was, I was not, I was, I was a little bit scared because I was afraid I was gonna die. Uh, it was, uh, in in New York, very close to my my my father (mother)*, uh, he ..I I was just going to ...I was having...I knew...I knew... and scared me half to death. Uh, I...I couldn't say what I was saying... by myself and I was getting scared because, still getting scared. I couldn't say hardly anything at that time."*

He is starting to ramble, so I redirect him. "So the ambulance came?" I ask.

"That's correct."

"And then what happened?"

"As soon as, now I was going faster and faster. The...the..(ambulance)* started to move, but I...I...I knew that I was starting to move away and the..in fact, as the .. I couldn't say what was going on at that time...*

Redirecting again, I ask, "What happened at the hospital?"

"They were moving, is..is..in the truck, not the car but... but...but ..the...

"Ambulance?" I supply.

"The amalence. And I was going. I didn't ...started disappear and open back and disappear and open at that time (Blacking out?)*. They...they, uh, I remember, came up again and I could see what was going on. There were several, uh, uh, pater...paters.. to explain..."*

"Doctors?" I ask.

"Doctors. There were four. I'm pretty sure it was a, it was a...a...a...doctor, a...a woman, and there were four men and they were looking at me and I was looking by the self, but I was starting to foggery (get foggy) again. And the doctor, uh, push my hand (shows injecting a needle into his arm) and I realize its, the doctor, the doctor must be pushing, uh, and that was it. That was the last time for one hell of a long time and I think, I think it was close to ...to dead and there was...I saw, and I nothing, nothing, absolutely all."

He has a vague image of Kathleen walking beside him in the hospital, (probably the trip to the MRI unit two days before he left Maimonides). He relates the ambulance ride to Kernan with Kathleen.

"And I think then I was, I was going out, droving (driving) with several people, driving up to from New York to uh...

"Kernan?" I offer.

"Kernan. The oddly, and there was nothing else, but, but, there's a lot of people would be amazed at how well I could see them, what was going on, the most thing that I was over in the uh, the doctor, not a doctor...

"The ambulance?" I offer.

"Yes, and it was along, it was roughly about two, two, about two...about a couple, about several..."

"Hours?" I supplied the word.

"Hours. I was driving, but nobody else was know but I could see it all of a sudden. Amazing, I was ...one of the things, was driving, up, high, (he motions that his bed is high in the back of the ambulance and he can see out the windows) although people, I guess could, where the car is, and they didn't know that I did, but I did. And I could see, driving, cars...cars, one, two, three. I could on this side, and I could look to (with) an eyes see what was going on, driving along. It's a beautiful day and people were looking at it (the ambulance) and I could see what, what was going on, and I passed out a little bit later."

Two weeks of lost memories. He has no recollection of visitors, no memory of Dr. Anant, no awareness of anything that happened to him at Maimonides. It's probably just as well, although I wouldn't have minded of he'd lied a little and said he remembered me too.

When he arrived at Kernan, he remembers knowing something was wrong with him, because there were nurses, but not being concerned about it.

He describes one very scary memory. He thinks it was his first or second night at Kernan. Much of the story he demonstrates. Lying alone in the dark, feeling naked, seeing no one, he feels clothes gently being placed over his body. His arms, which he cannot move, are then crossed over his chest, as if he is being prepared for burial. In his mind, this ceremonial rite, for that is what he perceives it to be, lasts for hours. He doesn't know if he is dying or already dead, but he is very much afraid. Suddenly the door to his room opens, flooding the room with light, a nurse enters and the image disappears. He believes she had rescued him from death. John describes this story to me partially in words and partially by his actions as I guess at the words and he confirms or denies them. In the past, he has only told me that he thought he had died, and I didn't understand what he meant. His communication has definitely improved. I wonder if it was a dream?

Of his therapists, he remembers two most fondly. Susan won him over the first day on the bicycle. Though her exercises for him got progressively harder each day, she was always careful and he trusted her completely. He held onto her, knowing he would fall if he did not, completely dependent on her to help him move. He never doubted that she could make him walk again, as long as he did what she said. He worked hard to recover, but he knew that Susan would make him walk again and he would be fine.

He remembers feeling that Janet, his OT, enjoyed being with him and helping him. She made him feel that being with him was the high point of her day. He says his time with her was fun and made him feel good about himself. What a wonderful gift she gave him!

Of the other therapists, he says they helped him to come back. And of me, he says that as long as we were together, he was "just fine". He remembers much of the work we did together, and of how eagerly he waited for my arrival each day.

He recalls one incident at Kernan with anger and frustration.

"I'm sitting there by by (my) *self. There are two doctors, uh, one I...I...I knew very well. The first time he'd ever been by this particular doctor* (the second) *... he started to talk to me and I knew exactly what what he was talking uh, but unfortunately, he cannot, the doctors cannot see. I can't say it and although can under...understand what my the the my doctor and I knew what was going on. Now it's different because I'm...I'm... I'm stupid...stupid. I...I...can't although I know what was going on, I couldn't say anything. The two doctors, they're both* (talking to) *me. The doctor would turn and would, and would say, would say fast, but I couldn't understand and I guess the trick is is that by myself, I have to think about it. And the way he would do it* (John speaks quickly and loudly), 'How do you...,What you don't..., What you do..., How can you..., Why can't you...Can't you..' That's exactly what he was saying. Although I could not say it, I have to think my myself. Although I could try to do it, I just couldn't do it. I could feel trying to hold on. It was like I was spart... smart, but I couldn't hold onto it. I really have to hold onto this. The doctor would say, 'Oh, he can't get it, he's, he's stupid, he can't do this, forget it, just drop him.' Although I could, I could thought it, I could most of it hold it, it would* (I was) *getting mad because one would turn to ...and say Ah, forget it, he can't understand, let's, let's forget it type-of-a-thing. And I feel very, uh, very terrible, although I knew everything what he was saying which would get mad* (me) *mad. Now there were two. One was relatively nice guy. I mean, he wouldn't really say it like that either. But one could make me like I'm stupid and it would make me so mad, but there's nothing I can do. Nothing bloody I can do."*

John's comprehension was apparently better than we realized. Even if he has an exaggerated or incorrect recollection of the situation, he clearly

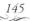

remembers the anger and frustration he felt at having questions asked more quickly than he could respond, at thinking that the doctor he did not know was talking about his lack of ability. Quite obviously, measuring what he could say was not a good way to measure what he could understand.

John was never aware of the jargon in his speech and occasionally listens in amazement at the recording taken two months after his stroke. He knew he couldn't always say what he wanted to say, but he expected it to get better and it didn't bother him. He thought he understood what was going on. In his mind he was okay. John spent most of his time around women, me, his therapists, his sisters, and he describes that as important with regard to how it made him feel more comfortable about talking.

"It's kind of odd thing, uh, number one, I liked people. I I just like it and I think it's because, more or less, a lot of people basically have helped me, and I'm sort of basically enjoint (enjoying) it for all sorts of reasons, because I'm looking and see what's going on. Give you an example. Women who just talk, particularly women, god, it's amazing how much people just bring what going on, and just, just say and you know I'm just looking (listening to) what's going on. Women seem to do that. Most women basically say what's going on so that I'm sort of interesting (interested) because, just for some reason, they talk. I'm always looking (listening) to what I'm enjoying. It seems that women, they're pretty doggone good. She helps what was going on, basically help. It's not that me, also is fine to do, but women, they constant talk back and forth, back and forth and its a help. Women are easier to help and all of a sudden, it's easier to talk."

John's remarks surprised me and I saw his positive attitude in a new light. To the extent that a person's opinion of himself is a reflection of the way people see him and treat him, John was treated, especially by the women around him, not only as if he was normal, but as if he was wonderful and special. In fairness, most of his time was spent around women. He liked being around people and he came away feeling just fine about himself. I always thought of depression as something that came from within, that no one else could control for us. Now I think more about how the world around us influences the way we feel. People can make us feel wonderful, can make life feel worth living. Barring clinical depression which requires medical intervention, treating people as if they are wonderful may make them wonderful. I keep learning from John.

This attitude explains a lot about why he didn't seem afraid, or angry, or depressed, but I think there's more. Loss and growth are both relative terms and at any given time, either could describe the same state.

One way I think of it is to imagine that there's a part of the brain that defines our universe. As we grow, our definition of the universe expands—we know more about ourselves, our capabilities, more about the world around us. As an adult, if we suddenly experience a great loss of many of our capabilities, like the ability to walk, or read, or write, or speak, we would expect to feel great sadness. Suddenly there is this great gap between our image of ourselves and our ability. One might understandably expect depression to set in. But an infant, learning to crawl, is happy with this new independence, not sad because he cannot yet walk. A toddler learning to walk is triumphant, not disappointed that he cannot run. When a child learns the alphabet, he is proud of his new skill, not depressed that reading is still beyond him. For a teenager learning to drive, the world expands again with this new freedom.

So it seemed with John. I believe the part of the brain that defined his universe was altered by his stroke in some strange way. His memory of the past was intact. Had his view of his universe shrunk to be consistent with his capabilities? Or was the part of his brain that should have told him about the terrible thing that happened broken? He says his brain protected him from what happened. He says that his brain got smaller, but it was full and he was okay. And it keeps getting bigger and that's full too. It's as if his brain feels no loss. So there is no sadness over a sense of loss, only joy as the brain continues to grow and redefine the universe. Each relearned skill expands his universe. And amazingly, the world from that perspective seems new and wonderful. Each new discovery is delightful, each achievement something to be proud of. He knows that he reads poorly, speaks with difficulty and can't write, so he is not in denial. It's just that he's not sad. He still expects to keep getting better, but he enjoys almost everything, and very little bothers him. He is still a driven person who works hard and is highly motivated. He says that he never feels unhappy. Honestly, I don't understand it. But I do know that I've only seen him sad a few of times, and then not for long.

More often, he views his communication problems as a challenge— almost a game that he enters into with relish. For example, he'll discover that he needs to buy something, like the attachment for the staple gun that lets you attach Christmas tree lights to the house. He can't find the one he used last year. First he must explain to me what he needs because I might know where it is. He can't say "staple" or "gun" or "attachment" or "lights", so the charades begin. He imitates stapling. I guess stapler. But he doesn't need a stapler. He wants me to go outside, but it's cold so I refuse, forcing him to move beyond the verbal impasse. He manages to say the word "lights" after several tries. I guess he wants to staple the lights onto the house. Does he need staples? No. He goes out to the garage and brings in a different kind of attachment. Does he need an attachment? Yes, but he can't find it. He draws a picture of the shape of the one he needs. Together we search the garage, but are unsuccessful, finding only the empty box that originally held it. He decides to go to the store. He has the empty box. He looks at me with an excited and challenged look on his face. "Do you think I can do it?" he asks with a grin. I begin to wonder if he lost it on purpose. He's having too much fun with this. And so it goes with each new hurdle. He thinks it's fun to solve the problem. Sometimes he asks me to write down what he needs, intending to use it only as a last resort, if he can't get it any other way. I once had a boss who said that there were no problems, only opportunities and challenges. John is the fulfillment of that statement.

And how am I? After surviving the terror of the first few days, I never tormented myself asking why this had happened to John, to us. Beyond the medical concern that we wanted to know if he was still in danger of a recurrence, there was no point in dwelling on the unfairness of it, and I felt no need to do so. My pity-party in the shower at Kathleen's house two days after the stroke, probably the lowest point in my life, was the last one I ever had or needed. My fear that I would not be able to do what had to be done was unfounded. In life, as in cards, you play with the hand that you have been dealt and though our hand looked terrible at first, we had the rest of our lives to win at this game. Our lives are forever changed. Our jobs are changed, but when I talk with friends about how much John had changed, they laugh and say how much I've changed too.

In the weeks following John's stroke, I felt an overwhelming need to have life return to normal without being able to define what that meant. Normal brought with it a certain predictability, a comfort level. The loss of it created a high level of confusion, uncertainty and anxiety. In a life unmarred by tragic events, where shifts occur gradually and changes are subtle, our concept of normal evolves over time, so gradually that we accept the changes without even acknowledging them. When a cataclysmic event occurs, we need time to distance ourselves from it, to see if it is just a blip on our radar, a temporary aberration, or whether it will forever alter our concept of normal. John's stroke shattered my former vision and left me fearful of the future, afraid that nothing would ever be the same again. In many ways it wasn't, but it is only in retrospect that I can see that it was at that moment in time, that pivotal instant that redefined the world we knew, when normal changed forever. And it is only later that I see that my definition of time changed too. I have discovered that I use a new time line to define events—"before John's stroke", "after John's stroke", as if the event that defines time is inextricably linked to the standard we apply to our vision of normal, as if that simple definition of time somehow explains all the life-altering effects that occurred at that moment. Life is normal again, but not the old normal. And this new standard for normal is certainly different, in some ways worse, in others better. But thank God, I feel normal again.

When I made the decision to close my company *Fastrak*, I questioned how I would spend all the hours in all the days for the rest of my life and what it would be like to be with John twenty-four hours a day. I wondered if I would grow to resent him. Well, we don't spend twenty-four hours a day together. I have been able to continue consulting locally on a limited basis, about forty days in 1999. In addition to providing income, I stay in contact with other professionals in my field. This arrangement has been ideal for me. John travels alone each Tuesday to Baltimore to meet with Charlotte, a good opportunity for him to contribute usefully to the community of research. We do much together, but also maintain separate interests and activities. We still read one to two hours every day. Weather permitting, John works in the yard most days. We can run errands together, or go separately. We take trips somewhere almost every month.

As John's independence grew, I became restless. I needed a new project. John was still my first priority but I wanted to do more. I often thought about writing a book, to share our experiences with other people in a way that would be helpful and informative. I remembered how difficult it had been when John had his stroke to find out what happened to other people in similar situations. Two days after John's surgery, I was searching for reading material. The technical books were there. The life stories were missing. I mentioned this idea to my sister Annie and was encouraged by her enthusiastic response.

This book is the product of that effort. I usually wrote during the day. Each night, John listened eagerly to new and revised passages. We laughed and cried many times together. Some things he remembers, some things surprise him, some he wants to hear over and over. He is my harshest critic, when he thinks something is confusing or just not right, and my strongest supporter. And so, boredom has not set in. Rather than resenting each other, we enjoy our time together and our time apart.

If someone had told me when I was twenty-one years old and a bright, ambitious college graduate, that I would someday be married to a man who had difficulty speaking, couldn't write and could barely read, I would have lived in dread, unable to believe that I wouldn't be miserable or resentful. Thank God we don't know the future. How could I have understood that those characteristics would not define the man? How could I, who placed so much importance in literacy and education, have believed that this man would be my great love? I could not have understood then, that while these characteristics limit John, they would never define him. This shift in values has changed me, redefined what is important, hopefully made me more tolerant, less judgmental, perhaps taught me more about patience, certainly opened my eyes to love.

Before John's stroke, I was so busy doing things that there wasn't much time or energy left for people. That has changed. Family has taken on a more important role. Several times a week I'm on the phone with family members, both John's and mine. I've discovered I really like John's family. We speak and visit often, especially with Kathleen, and laugh a lot. My sons call at least weekly just to talk, not because they need money, and actually ask my opinion about things. Have they grown up or have I? Loving John, and telling him, has made it easier for me to tell my boys I love them too. I always loved them, it just wasn't something I said very often. Now I feel comfortable saying it. I wish I could have before. My family is closer too. We see each other more often, talk frequently, and share our feeling more. I didn't know how much I was missing.

When I think of John, I think of a man who cheerfully gets up every morning and works hard all day. I see a man who is honest, kind, generous and thoughtful. I think of a man with a great sense of humor, who spends a lot of time laughing, at himself, at me, and at the idiosyncrasies of everyday life. This is a man for whom I have an incredible amount of admiration, respect and pride. How many of us really work to be all that we can be? Everyday, I feel his hugs and hear his words of love. We are now physically more affectionate, emotionally more involved and committed, and intellectually very challenged. I know now that labels may describe, but don't define people. Somehow, we're just so very right together. I guess what surprises me most is how happy we are.

I should also mention that some of John's "less wonderful" traits have begun to emerge. As his independence has grown, and his confidence in making decisions increases, he is more vocal about what he does and doesn't want to do. He's less willing to "go along for the ride", more likely to say he doesn't want to do something, quicker to criticize. His dislike for window-shopping has reemerged. And sometimes, yes, even John can be unreasonable. I get really irritated when he refuses to run an extra errand when we are already out, instead, expecting me to make a separate trip to do it. When I put it in perspective, I call it "getting better", wondering if he is becoming more "left-brained" again, but I don't always enjoy it. Thank God for love.

One late afternoon in May of 1999, shortly after arriving at the home of a favorite couple of ours, Noel and Diana who lived outside Denver, John and Noel wandered into the den on the "guy's version" of the house tour. Diana and I were catching up in the kitchen, having seen little of each other in the past few years.

Diana remarked, "John looks wonderful. He's doing so well and he seems so happy. It's like a miracle. When I think of you, I think of all the sacrifices you made for John."

I was silent for a few seconds. I hadn't thought about the word "sacrifice" for a long time, not since the first few days after John's stroke. Had I sacrificed anything?

"I don't think I made any sacrifices for John. I don't feel like I have. I always did exactly what I wanted to do, I made every choice freely. In the beginning, right after John's stroke, I was afraid my life might be over. I worried about whether I could sacrifice my life for John. I wasn't sure I was willing to do it. But it never turned out to be an issue. When you do what you want to do, how can that be sacrifice? Actually, it feels rather selfish."

Sacrifice, it turned out, was never an issue.

I know a lot more about strokes than I did three years ago, both because of the people we've met and the reading we've done. I've learned how different every person's stroke is and each new story amazes and inspires me. I also know how fortunate we were that John had disability insurance and we were financially able to live comfortably without having to work to support ourselves. We feel blessed by so many of the circumstances surrounding our lives, the support of family and friends, John's remarkable physical recovery, his wonderful positive attitude.

It is still relatively early in his stroke recovery to know what the future holds for him, for us, but the hard work of recovery will continue. And we shall continue to pray for the miracles.

The eleven o'clock news has just ended. Already in bed, John turns off the TV and lowers the dimmer switch on the overhead light.

I whisper, "Good night sweetheart, I love you."

"I love you too."

We fall asleep, snuggled up together, spoon-style under the covers.

If success is a journey, then we're on our way. John is the most successful man I have ever met and I'm the luckiest woman. I thank God that life goes on.

List of Characters

Alice	Kathleen's daughter in Brooklyn
Allison	John's speech therapist after returning home
Annie and Jeff	Eileen's sister in Maryland and her brother-in-law
Art	A long time friend of John
Brendan	John's brother in Dubuque
Charlotte Mitchum	Researcher at University of Maryland Medical Center
Christopher	John's son in Salt Lake City
David	Eileen's son in Maryland
Dr. Anant	The neurosurgeon who performed the craniotomy
Dr. LaMonte	John's specialist after he returned home
Dr. Makley	John's doctor at Kernan
Eileen	John's wife, the author
Janet	John's daughter in Maryland
Janet	John's occupational therapist at Kernan
Jeanne	Brendan's wife
Jeannie	Kathleen's daughter in Brooklyn
John	The stroke survivor
John Andrew	John's son in Las Vegas
Kathleen	John's sister in Brooklyn
Mary and Steve	John's sister in Manhattan and his brother-in-law
Paul	Eileen's brother in Houston
Richard	Eileen's brother in Toronto
Roger	Long time friend of John
Sean	Eileen's son in Albuquerque
Susan	John's physical therapist
Thomas	Kathleen's son in Brooklyn